FITLOSOPHY

BY SOPHIE THOMAS

Printed in the United States of America
Print ISBN: 978-1-956019-25-4
eBook ISBN: 978-1-956019-26-1

Library of Congress Control Number: 2021921912

Published by DartFrog Blue, the traditional
publishing imprint of DartFrog Books.

Publisher Information:
DartFrog Books
4697 Main Street
Manchester, VT 05255
www.DartFrogBooks.com

Join the discussion of this book on Bookclubz. Bookclubz
is an online management tool for book clubs, available
now for Android and iOS and via Bookclubz.com.

For my friends and family, and for any of those who have endured my esoteric ramblings and harebrained theories on utilising philosophy for a better life.

WHY PHILOSOPHY?

Back in my sixth-form days, I was what you'd definitely label a loser. I had very few friends, and this was purely exacerbated by the various depressive and anxious episodes I encountered over the years.

This isn't to garner pity or sympathy: rather, it's indicative of how and why the ideas and theories and wisdom of those giants before me helped reframe suffering, struggling, and the general mediocrities of daily living.

A dull, nauseous shadow would shimmer beyond daybreak's horizon as I slumped out of bed. How could I attempt social niceties feeling like this? What even was the point of existing where I felt totally useless, without purpose or goals or striving?

A caveat before I continue: dusty tomes and wise adages are not the panacea to mental illness. The only way I managed to deal, and still to this day deal, with my condition was through professional help, medication, and the irrevocable love and support I have been surrounded with. They have, however, acted as a massive catalyst for mindful introspection and coping mechanisms to design my own lifestyle and become a person who I'd quite like to become.

Now that you've gotten some idea of how much of an awkward creature I was mentally and emotionally, you'll get a real crack out of the purported physical prowess of a so-called personal trainer.

A game of rounders threw me into (even more) existential despair. I could hardly run a bath, let alone run. And I'd regularly pretend that I was "on my period" to get out of PE class. I think by the time I left school, my teachers must've assumed something was seriously wrong with my uterus.

Around this time, I was also, for better or for worse, getting into modelling. There appears to be very little, if any, correlation to philosophy in this current trajectory, but hang in there, the rambling will soon cease, and you'll all be liberated.

Modelling gave me a lot of things—some good, some bad. A dose of crippling, chronic self-doubt and the incessant ache of inferiority complex. All excellent components to ease my depression, as you can outrightly see.

But it did give me a sense of belonging, a jolt of extraversion and adaptation when I could only be best described as a very sad and a very lonely hermit crab, except a hermit crab who still hadn't found its forever shell. And as all hermit crabs must inevitably feel when coasting from shell to shell, I felt pretty bereft, which I'd wager is normal in the tumultuous period of adolescence, but at the time, like any dolefully narcissistic youth, I prioritised feeling like I could "find myself"—whatever the hell that meant or means.

Thus being able to chat to quirky photographers about their cacti collection in a rundown East London apartment-cum-studio or be buffeted by plush, foundation-drenched brushes and empty compliments enabled me to find a temporary shelter in the form of the fashion industry. If that were a shell, I have no literal clue what it'd look like. Perhaps some kind of flamboyant conch, peddled with glitter or florals or pretentious monochrome, something that wouldn't look amiss if an artist put it up for exhibition at the Tate.

Anyway, that was my shell. As flimsy and superficial and meaningless as it ultimately was.

There were a few sturdy barnacles attached to what seems a purely empty experience. I learnt the meaning of setting up and keeping boundaries, even as a sixteen-year-old. My empathy levels were exacerbated by seeing other people around me be eviscerated by the same designer or casting director or gossip magazine. And I really did learn that all this "stuff" was ephemeral at best and poisonous at worst. Whilst I still model today, it's nowhere near as much of a priority. I finally took it off that pedestal it lounged upon for many years and tucked it neatly away in my souvenir box, taking it out occasionally to give it a good sheen or take what I need from it, and nothing more.

If you ask me, it looks much better there than it ever did centre stage.

What wasn't impermanent, and what still remains my main prize on show, was the catalyst I gained for training and exercising and overhauling my lifestyle.

Granted, at first, it was purely superficial, a menial chore done in the name of booking jobs and appeasing haughty clients. At that point, it felt like I was being played by a very green and very overcooked actor, and the real Sophie was a thousand miles away, living an integrity-filled life I had aspired to but could somehow never really grasp, like wisps of mists between my fingers, fizzling out in the sunrise.

But that hour of movement or training or just pure *escape* became something so much more than part of my day job. It became a harbinger of change and renewal. Introspection and consideration. Triggering questions like who I wanted to be and how I'd get there in the end. I was suffering from enormous depressive episodes and was stuck in a ditch of suicidal ideation, self-harming, and feeling isolated and alone from the rest of my loved ones. This was around nine-odd years ago, and I can clearly see the demarcated difference in mental health discussion then versus now. Granted, we have ways to go, but there has been more openness. There has been more admittance and acceptance, and although this sounds awfully solipsistic and n=1-like, from personal experience, the variance in how my friends and family respond to a self-confessed mental health dip is like night and day.

At the best of times, I'm terrible at physical calisthenics and actual gymnastics (long, hyper-mobile limbs and dyspraxia should not ever twain) but my mental gymnastics, in case you couldn't tell from this loquacious, overt introduction, is top-notch.

From the processing of how I felt by taking charge of my life-style and making small, beneficial differences to the way I live and how I wanted to improve myself, I saw a correlation with phi-losophy and the way many great thinkers, past and present, saw the need to cultivate one's own inner garden as a way to pursue a fortuitous, fruitful life.

It got me questioning not just the basis of existence—a nice little mental pre-ambling before breakfast time, of course—but what it meant to lead a good life, to be a decent individual, and how the betterment of oneself, physically and mentally, entailed that by ex-tension we could help support and ameliorate the roots of society. By how we think, by how we act, and by how we choose to simply be.

I started exploring and seeing this in not only a broader, societal sense but well within the microcosmic realm of health and fitness. Which sounds ludicrous, I know. And I think only someone with the daft and vast skills of mental gymnastics, such as me, could come up with something so profoundly obsolete. But it was damn fun to look at and has proven to be even more fun to create as part of a project. It has also enabled me to better understand myself, my clients, and how to tailor each approach to their goals appropriately and in a way that lauds better rates of success. Taken with a massive pinch of salt, of course—the true, unashamed pursuit of this has been to encourage people to question the narrative, learn about old wisdom and tricky ethical arguments, and hopefully make philosophy somewhat palatable. Because I will be the first to admit it can get dry. *Real* dry.

OKAY, GREAT.
BUT WHY FITLOSOPHY?

This brings me on to formatting my ideas into one silly conglomerate: a pseudo-personality test known as Fitlosophy. Like most personality tests out there, it is invariably highly flawed: for one, personality is not some static, paralysed construct, and even models such as the Big Factor Five have had some of the more rigorous scrutinies in terms of study replication has its issues. For instance, only a few of the traits it measures have significant test-retest, examined in a forty-five-year test-retest period. This infers that the test fails to account for the research now pointing out, more than ever, that personality structure can change throughout the whole lifespan. There are also raised concerns about how some of the traits have underlying environmental and genetic determinants, which likely becomes a methodological flaw. There also does not appear to be adequate coverage in the Factor Five Model for psychotic traits, so whilst it may not be directly helpful for psychiatric diagnosis, it may still capture heterogeneity within diagnostic criteria.

Fitlosophy shares these and many other problems: in a nutshell, it's a bit of fun to help you best identify with how you prefer to tackle goals and fitness quandaries, all dressed up as light-hearted edutainment in an attempt to make philosophy (at least, somewhat) enjoyable.

But you can imagine, seeing as such a well-thought-out and critiqued personality test such as Cattell's has its fair share of problems, that this little archetype test from a philosophy lover will have a plethora of methodological issues.

In short: whilst this is to be taken with a massive pinch—nay, bucket-load—of salt, it is in good faith and fun and will hopefully get you to better understand yourself a little bit in addition to the way you train, the way you behave, and the way you think.

Its aim is also to promote critical, lateral thinking in the form of looking at the various (albeit diluted) philosophical theories before you and encourage more reading on a certain topic, or get you interested in a certain thinker or way of discussion that may best appeal to you.

It's vital to remember that in philosophy, there are no "good" or "bad" arguments, really, unless you're discussing morality (and even then, those terms aren't especially used), but it's best to look at arguments through a "valid" or "sound" lens. We'll be going over these terms in due course.

It's very normal and natural for us to find a tribe or community, so to speak, that harkens to our own needs and worldviews. As humans, we are natural storytellers and listeners to stories, and just as we are drawn or repelled by certain films or books or genres, so too will we have our own personal preferences in all walks of life. The richness and complexity of our own genetics, childhood experiences, interpersonal relationships, and even varied exposure to sociological phenomena will contribute to the formatting of opinion, behaviour, and even personality.

New research, however, pinpoints adult personality and behaviour as being slightly mutable and not as static as we once assumed it to be. This is exciting news in the realm of psychology. It throws into the question the a priori assumption that once you've experienced a trauma or been brought up in a puritanical, conservative family setting or had a shitty ex, then that was it—your brain structure adapted to suit the needs of these circumstances. It questions those personality tests that once assumed a trait was a trait, static and solid and unencroachable. But we are slowly beginning to see that there is much more nuanced than first presumed.

There are worlds within us all, and we are the gods: there is a modicum of input that we are able to contribute through what we do, read, and who we read and speak to, for instance. And there will always be a type of thinking that might draw us in or a biological urgency underpinning a certain habit. There is some structural and biopsychological engineering that is unavoidable, or at least manageable at the very most. But that does not mean we cannot expose ourselves and be open to other opinions, ways of thinking, or approaches to certain issues. We can navigate the at times tumultuous oceans of nervous-system response and learn for different ideas and viewpoints to cohabit our inner universe at once without imploding violently.

Fitlosophy, in one part, is to assign you better guidance to tackle your goals, yes. But it is a hope of mine that it will also encourage you to read and relish different opinions without recoiling or assuming it questions your own set of values or personally ascribed communities. I want you to be able to take all these different approaches and decide for yourself what argument sits best with you and why. I want you to hopefully become more cognisant of arguments that smell a bit off, to be more aware of unscrupulous people trying to sell a lie, and understand that the framework of morality, although one that has been contested for centuries is of utmost importance to discuss. I want you to love *thinking*.

KARL MARX AND THE MARXIST FITLOSOPHER

One of the most influential political philosophers out there, you'd be hard-pressed to find somebody who *hasn't* heard of this famous, bearded revolutionary. Karl Marx (1818–1883) is best known for his economic and historical analysis in his writings, coming up with a concept known as *dialectical materialism*, and his ideas have been the foundation for social and political change even now. Marx has written swathes and swathes on political philosophy, so for this section on Fitlosophy, we'll be focusing on one particular concept that gets parroted out a lot (often, incorrectly) by anyone politically engaged. Additionally, it appears to be the term most applicable for our endeavouring Fitlosophers.

First, let's try and clarify by what he means when he uses the term dialectical materialism. Marx uses a lot of specific terminologies, which may mean it can be very tricky getting our head around the actual core content of his philosophies and understanding them in an applicable way.

So, it's best to start with one of the better-known terms. Marx based this idea on Hegel's analysis of history. In Hegelian philosophy (although Hegel is bloody horrible to read and study so you can imagine why I have chosen to leave him out of Fitlosophy) «dialectical" is a term here that refers to some kind of conversation or conflict or debate. Hegel applied this to understanding human history through the course of the ages: he figured that historical proceedings were actually a manifestation of what he dubbed the "spirit" (in his words, zeitgeist) of a certain epoch.

Now, let's say Hegel was trying to study the '40s (if he was a historian today.) He would argue that the «zeitgeist" or fundamental spirit of this era would be fighting against all that was known about the 20s, as an example. Prohibition was fought against, and the Second World War brought in substantial political and sociological change compared to the somewhat cavalier nature of the '20s. Hegel argued that this clashing of timelines would then bring about a *synthesis*—otherwise known as a new age, culminating from this constant back and forth from eras. As a result, Hegel hypothesised that the ultimate form of truth would arrive to humanity to the end of all of this historical squabbling.

I know this isn't exactly Marxist philosophy, but trust me, I haven't scammed you (yet); learning about Hegel is imperative to understanding Marx's own thoughts and applying it to our own everyday practice.

In some ways, Hegel's dialectic also makes it easier for us to view tragic occurrences and historical upheaval, as, through his logic, we can interpret it as being a natural path of the course if we are to fully realise a greater future. What do *you* think?

Marx was inspired by Hegel and took a lot from his work. This time, however, instead of purely fixating on the development of history, Marx applied the concept of the dialectic to what we dub the material: that includes money, goods, and general economic resources. By applying the dialectic in such a way, he noticed a large disparity between classes: the middle or higher classes, which he labelled the Bourgeoisie, had a vast collection of resources in comparison to the working classes, named the proletariat. This was especially important as during Marx's life, there was an upheaval in industrialisation, including factories, and the rise of corporate planning, which made Marx's observation all the more stark.

But where does the concept of historical «zeitgeist" or spirit come into play now? Hegel's concept of the dialectic was an abstract one, in that he was describing different eras interplaying and conflicting with one another until the truth revealed itself. For Marx, this is manifested in the way goods and resources are shared and traded amongst ourselves and became a class conflict between those who had more material goods and resources versus those who did not. Marx defined these «age spirits" by different stages revolving around economic concerns and classist concepts.

- The first historical zeitgeist, according to Marx, would be manifested through the lens of Feudalism, essentially a system of monarchs and peasants. We can see examples of this scattered throughout the political system during the fifth and fifteenth centuries.
- The opposite of this zeitgeist emerges thereafter and is one we are all familiar with: Capitalism. Marx described this as ownership of goods—or the means of production—by the Bourgeoisie.
- Theoretically, Marx describes this conflict between the two ideologies as birthing the lovechild we know as Communism,

whereby the goods are shared, and people take according to their needs and contribute according to their ability.

Marx decided to build up a more concrete and material understanding of the dialectic: as opposed to merely examining timeframes and historical periods, he attempts to seek an understanding as to how humans behave, interact, exchange resources, and live and work together.

In short: in terms of philosophy, Marx was a materialist. Some thinkers are what we know to be called **idealists**, which essentially try to posit consciousness above everything else. (Ironically named, I know.) Materialism, however, is the view that everything—including consciousness—may be explained by material processes.

If we are to apply an analysis of history, for instance, an idealist might focus on the ideas and moralities of a certain age, arguing that these are the factors that have shaped that particular period of history. Marx would counter this, stating that ideas and the like certainly don't come from anywhere, and notes that these ideas are actually shaped by tangible, measurable processes we can see: class factions, economic distribution, and property laws, for example.

But How in Fresh Hell Does Rebelling Against the Bourgeoisie Add to My Fitness Levels?

Like Marx views the explanation of historical events as a material process, fitness dialectical materialism will see a goal or a journey in the same way: measurable, tangible, and summarised by the material, empirical evidence set before us.

Dialectical materialism in terms of fitness will prioritise the staples to achieving success in fitness. Calorie and macro tracking, progressive overload, and ardently physical, concrete outcomes are what one might fixate upon if this is the Fitlosophy that best suits their approach.

As a side: the praxis and social critique that Marx enlisted upon his readers and workers of the world has still infiltrated into a health skepticism toward corporatism today. Knowing when to call out the fitness industry on its capitalistic, vampiric elements is essential if we want to improve it, and we can only do so by being aware of the material conditions that create such settings in the first place.

The Marxist Fitlosopher

A Marxist Fitlosopher will, whether client or coach, partake in an evidence-based approach to the nth degree. You'll set forth material conditions in order for success to take place. You'll likely be a stickler for set routines, such as certain grams of protein per meal, sleeping times, and even tracking rest times to the last millisecond. There might be a slight correlation between Marxist Fitlosophers and those who frequent the land of strength and conditioning. The reason for this is thus: you are cognisant of the material conditions required to obtain a degree of success in improving physical prowess and will stick to it.

The question is, how can we define such parameters if we are to measure success? And how can we review, in the same way Marx did with historical events, the conflicts between fitness ideology and fitness ideology in such a way that we arrive at the 'ultimate truth'?

We're unlikely to meet it anytime soon, suffice to say. And a Marxist Fitlosopher might be aware of this and may express skepticism and protest at both quackery and corruption littered across the industry.

If these phrases feel familiar to you, you might appreciate, or naturally lean toward, the materialist approach in your goal setting:

- "Eat, sleep, lift. That's the way to go. Keep it simple, follow the rules."
- "Calories in, calories out. Simple as that, I'll eat a little bit less, and it should be good to go."
- "I don't really see food anymore; I just see my macro split on a plate."

However, a Marxist Fitlosopher will be the first one to investigate. They'll be trawling through research papers, assigning themselves to the mast of evidence-based physical activity. For example, a coach aware of the physiological conditions of fat loss might naturally espouse solutions for the issue of maintaining a calorie deficit whilst eschewing viewpoints that argue for a more holistic viewpoint or denote that there are contributing factors to a person's dietary intake. Like how a Marxist philosopher would argue that the material conditions, be it economic, class-related, or regarding the disparity of wealth, are the driving factors toward historical ideas, concepts, and motifs, the Marxist Fitlosopher would argue that calorie intake and regularly progressive overloads are the underpinning factor to obtaining better, holistic health and mental wellbeing. In a sense, they may see these factors as part of the cause-and-effect paradigm. You could argue that this debate is similar to how we start incessantly nattering over whether the chicken or the egg came first; for some, the egg is what creates the population of the chickens in the first place, whereas others argue without a chicken, there can be no egg for this growth to continue.

It may be possible that as a Marxist Fitlosopher, you tend to look through your own fitness journey as one that is purely empirical and quantitative. If we are to read the works of Marx and other materialist philosophers, we might find that the writing style is an outright match for their views: economical, concise, and hardly poetic. There's no real room for metaphysical interpretation in the same way you'll find in a piece of writing about consciousness, for instance. The discussion is mostly confined (and I certainly do not mean this as an insult) to material circumstances, which in essence was Marx's goal to outline the tragic inequalities and issues facing a brave new world, inundated with industrialisation without particularly knowing how to fare with it. Similarly, a Marxist Fitlosopher may be fixated on what is tangible and what is known; a sensible outlook considering both nutrition and sports science is relatively young branches in the behemoth of scientific flora.

It might be more likely you look toward methodological habits to achieve a certain outcome. Rather than weighing up the whys and ho's of not being able to reach a certain goal or musing upon the thousands of implications to how that is, you'll likely just crack on and see it as another day. Being driven by this evidence-based approach and *trusting* that the outcome will transpire if certain procedures are followed can be somewhat mirrored in the way Marx interpreted the rise and fall of feudalistic and capitalistic eras: it's using what you know, based on history and evidence and the conditions you can measure, and trying to come up with an outcome that best suits these frameworks.

In short, you're likely a stickler for the rules and reasonings postulated by the giants of the industry. Your Instagram «following" list might resemble more of a research paper references section than a social media application. This sets you up for a darn good precedent to mistrust fitness fables and get on with the dirty work required to obtain the outcome you desire.

Nonetheless, applying such a quantitative outlook regarding health and fitness goals may become slightly problematic for your own sanity. There are a fair few reasons for this, and they boil down to the fact that carving out a regimen for yourself, whether you're a total exercise newbie or training for your next triathlon, requires some sort of behaviour or habit change. And behaviour change in human beings is inexorably tricky and unpredictable.

And therein lies the issue with relying on research papers with select sample size and minimal impact factor: by solely looking at the human being as a fleshy bag of meaningless atoms, we forget the other factors that contribute to our self-actualisation and achievements. In a similar vein, some may argue Marx, despite his rigorous and articulate rhetoric, misses some of the more introspective questions that are in and of themselves difficult to quantify.

It's salubrious and sensible to follow guidelines backed by science and trust the process. The issue is not the ingredients required to get to your outcome, but rather the fact that often, said ingredients come without a set of instructions to create the recipe you want.

Humans are richly mangled messes, confounding complexities, and reducing our needs and desire and hopes and dreams and worldviews and experiences, good and bad, sorely miss out on creating a bespoke approach for you when it comes to achieving your fitness goals.

Let's take, for example, the (perfectly valid and true) statement that in order for us to lose weight, we must be in a caloric deficit. This is 100 percent true, and I have no contestation with this claim. Moreover, it is the grey area, the minute implications, that we must watch out for. There might be, for example, an individual who has suffered tremendous trauma and issues with food and eating in general. This individual looks at this statement without so much of an additional guideline to stipulate how to achieve said calorie deficit and embarks upon a journey of either tracking or counting or assuming higher-calorie content foods to be "bad" or "not allowed."

Are they following this statement truly and correctly? Technically, yes. Will they lose weight? We have no idea. The potential issues with such an individual's battered self-esteem and confusion surrounding food confound this issue. Rather than finding sustainability in consuming chicken and greens, day-in and day-out, they become so fixated on their body image and may develop, at best, an emotionally exhausting relationship with food or, at worst, another disorder.

If we are to assume said individual manages to soothe any triggers or painful emotions that do come up and avoids this treacherous path to relapse and does indeed lose the weight, on paper, it appears as if this methodology has succeeded. Numbers and data don't lie, after all, and this is perfectly quantifiable. These are, indeed, material and concrete and strong evidence of this individual's success in achieving a certain goal.

But does it mention their happiness? What they learnt? Any personal growth? Any long-term tweaks to said goal? Does it mention how or if they managed to heal any aspects of themselves in regards to control, body image, or eating?

The issue with reducing our goals and needs to numbers is thus: we simply cannot cultivate any more purpose beyond that of the stipulated target by any means necessary. Indeed, Marx warns that revolution, no matter how raucous, is violent and warranted per his prediction, based on the evidence that the material conditions have given him.

Humans are far more complex than what is suggested by small fragments of data. Therefore, we must take this into account—alongside the verifiable, falsifiable science, if we are to have a healthy and sustainable outlook on achieving any given goal.

How Can a Marxist Fitlosopher Find Balance?

More likely than not, if you tend to err on the side of this approach to fitness and health, then odds are, you have a pretty good grasp on aiming for a logical and sensible approach. You're probably happy with your methodologies and how you get from A to B. And there's a good chance you understand and appreciate the nuance of human beings, and don't let the maladaptive habits of black and white thinking interrupt your goals.

If, however, you're struggling to pursue a balance of focusing on the concrete and tangible with accepting some of your humanity, then it might get a little tricker. You might blame yourself or even others if you end up unsuccessful in achieving a goal. You might end up in a behavioural loop, repeating similar habits and actions fruitlessly without pausing to consider tweaking strategies. You may even find yourself fixated on the end goal without thinking about *how* to get there.

This, my friends, is where a little bit of metaphysical philosophy comes in. Just a touch.

As we've discussed before, Marx was never a fan of pursuing the knowledge of the abstract. This means you'll be hard-pressed to discover much on morality or being or time or space. He believed that a worthwhile philosophical pursuit was only in the material, as it offered us a more useful scope for understanding human behaviour. Marx was an immensely clever man, but personally, this is where I believe his argument's flaws are particularly enhanced.

As neuropsychological evidence is unpacking, it is evident that human behaviour and their condition itself is far more complex than just a set of genomes or a ploy of purely environmental factors. It's perfectly healthy and arguably more beneficial to say we just don't know everything yet. Sometimes it's better to admit the shortcomings of a solely allopathic route rather than die on a hill needlessly and, in this case, hungrily.

If you find your materialist leanings are affecting the way you interpret how you behave, for example, it might be worth taking a step back and considering the psychological and sociological implications behind the way you eat and form habits before breaking down squat mechanics or macro splits.

Understanding the whys and hows of human behaviour can lean into quantitative, subjective discussions—which is no bad thing, even if Marx contests this. Considering a greater purpose in your training, for example, is absolutely not a materialist perspective but a truly important one. "Wanting to lose weight" may not be your bottom line, for example. If we dig deeper and refine that desire, that dream, it might look a bit more like "feel more confident around my friends and help alleviate my social anxiety." Everyone's greater "why" is different, and to uncover hidden treasure may require some serious digging into darker depths you've kept locked up tight and discreet and safely tucked away. It may be painful. But discovering a more substantial meaning to your original game plan will most likely yield a more sustained, bespoke plan.

The biopsychosocial model is something that we'll touch upon more in this project, as I find it's fully relevant to taking a better glimpse into the way we act and behave. Like most theories, it still has its flaws—its replicability can be murky, and it's far easier to generate research based on biomedical approaches—but I believe once the data crisis in psychology begins to ease, we'll discover more interesting findings nonetheless.

This model was first proposed in 1977 by George Engel, a psychiatrist who grew weary of treating his patients like flesh and numbers and realised there was more to treating a complex human being. He believed that the biological should not only be the main thing we consider when it comes to health but also psychological and social factors. The psychological may include something like how an individual processes an experience or internalises their emotions. For instance, somebody may be more predisposed to experiencing depressive episodes or anxious preoccupations compared to another. Likewise, the sociological factor is vitally important (and arguably could fit in well with a Marxist approach, in any case) as it showcases the political, financial, personal, and systemic structures that surround an individual and form a part of their lives, for better or for worse.

There will be many instances when a more concrete answer is necessary. There's no doubt that if you're more of a Marxist Fitloso-pher, you're a whizz at deconstructing toxic myths or breaking down poor arguments that hold little to no water in the realm of research.

But there may also be times when this becomes black and white thinking. You might even become snarky and dismissive to other more holistic approaches—approaches that try to encapsulate non-quan-titative concepts like mood or emotion or daily stress levels.

All to say: the Marxist Fitlosopher need not detract from their own pool of knowledge or evidence-based approach but take into consideration the whole picture and not just the concrete writings you see before you.

If you find yourself engaging in these "upper extremities" of be-haviours, it might be best for you to take a step back and consider what this attitude offers you in daily living.

We want to get to the root of why there's safety and ease in choosing the black and white route. We can then see the benefits of sticking to the view and its costs.

Behaviour/worldview	Benefit	Cost
"Calories in, calories out. That's the best thing to focus on."	1. Concrete and tangible. 1. Evidence-based and the route to weight loss. 2. Easy instructions to follow; clear-cut and simple.	2. Negates psychological aspect of calorie deficit. 1. Might be difficult to sustain with little motive behind the statement. 2. Fails to take into account emotional aspect of lifestyle change.
"Progressive overload is the best way to get fitter."	7. A fixed, concentrated route on strength work and accumulating more muscle. 8. Ensures that you track your sessions diligently and view your progress. 9. Evidence-based and provides a decent base for power and speed development in sport.	1. Ignores skill development and biomechanics above the sacred gospel of S&C. 1. Runs the risk of not exercising or moving for joy in addition to pragmatic sessions— could create burnout or stale relationship with exercise. 1. "Best way" is reductive and overlooks the fact people have different preferences and goals.

By doing this table, we can start to see there is a sweet spot—a space for both the overtly rationalist and quasi-qualitative. A place where we can reconcile our own beliefs, biases, and research preferences and the overarching values for human growth and potential actualisation, the latter of which is inexorably difficult to replicate in lab settings, yet remains a prominent feature of society as a whole and how we navigate ourselves in that space.

The Marxist Fitlosopher can also challenge their black and white thinking if it becomes vociferous. This is important when interacting with others and being able to hold a different opinion on research or approaches whilst maintaining composure and decorum. A good example of this not taking place is generally surrounding activities such as CrossFit, a collective experience which undoubtedly has its issues in specificity and values, yet still holds huge merit in cultivating community and support as opposed to an individualistic gym setting. It is likely (and often the case) that examples such as CrossFit attract the candour and snark across the industry, referred to as cult-like or bro science.

Whether these statements are truly false remains to be seen, but its importance in these claims is immediately washed away and potentially invalidates an individual's hugely positive experience in regards to mental health or self-confidence. It may therefore be prudent for the Marxist Fitlosopher to learn to sit with differing views and approaches in a way that still validates their own experience whilst honouring the lifestyles of others—provided that those lifestyles are not harming that individual or others around them.

ARISTOTLE AND THE ARISTOTELIAN FITLOSOPHER

Aristotle will be one of the names in this series that you'll have likely heard of, and for a good reason: in terms of philosophy, Aristotle is considered one of the proprietors of Western logic and was one of the heavyweights in the realm of ancient Greece. Current thinkers should be thankful for this man's contributions, as he helped formulate a rationale and way of breaking down arguments into coherent, valid forms.

Aristotle often took part in the use of *syllogistic reasoning*. His aim was essentially to walk the thinker through a prediction, from hypothesis all the way to a summary or conclusion. A basic idea of what Aristotle did with these syllogisms would be something like this:

If 1 is predictive of all 2,
And 2 is predictive of all 3,
Then 2 is predictive of all 3.

When we are aware of the premises and are able to make conclusions from following said premises, Aristotle asserts that we gain knowledge by practicing this logic of debate and discussion. We need to basically be practical about going from premise to conclusion if we are to attain a status of validity of these premises.

His creation of logic and causal reasoning forms a framework for most of his general thinking, but what makes Aristotle different from someone more black and white such as Marx, is that he acknowledges the possibility of knowledge not being some static, purely empirical concept. Rather, he explores and recognises the existence of metaphysical concepts and endeavours to dive into them. Ethics, for instance, is one such topic that he is incredibly well-known for and delves into it splendidly. One of his most famous views, found in the work *Nicomachean Ethics*, postulates that we are able to achieve excellence—a term he defines as being virtuous and a sort of happiness—through practice and coherent behaviours that match with a set of values. He called this state of blissful, meaningful living *eudaimonia,* another famous term you may have heard scattered about the realms of non-philosophy.

Through his formation of logic and proposal of purposeful living, Aristotle's ideas are widely associated with concepts such as self-improvement, lifestyle change, and discipline over hedonism. Thus, it only seems appropriate that we slot him into this series. For the sake of being concise—a task that is hard enough as it is for my loquacious tendencies—we will be studying his use of eudaimonia and how it correlates to Fitlosophers who embark down this path of habit and behaviour change.

Aristotle's commentary on different subjects and issues runs far and wide without compromising breadth. It goes without saying, considering the terms we have just discussed, like "virtuous," "happiness," "excellence," and "values," Aristotle was unlike Marx in that he favoured discussion of the intangible and metaphysical as he believed it acts as a forebear to the practical and material. In Aristotle's works, eudaimonia was (based on older Greek tradition) used as the term for the highest human good, and so it is the aim of practical philosophy, including ethics and political philosophy, to consider (and also experience) what it really is, and how it can be achieved. In *Nicomachean Ethics*, Aristotle also appears to reject that the highest good is God-given, which is a useful rebuttal for those who espouse that metaphysical discussion resides solely for the religiously inclined.

Aristotle divvied up these concepts into theoretical and practical philosophy. As the name suggests, theoretical philosophy implies contemplation and a greater understanding of metaphysical issues, whilst practical philosophy is centred on Aristotle's idea of contributing to and building upon the good life. Metaphysical and intangible discussions are necessary, however, for this part to flourish: Aristotle considered humans to be "political animals"— complex, variable, and too nuanced to be categorised into simplistic forms. Ethical inquiry, therefore, was necessary, according to Aristotle, to further investigate what leading a good life meant and how that would look in daily living.

As Aristotle proposes that ethics, values, and virtues are concepts to be put into practice, it only makes sense that an Aristotelian Fitlosopher would follow suit in the way they lead their lives and pursue their goals. Rather than assuming good habits or a specific outcome to happen rather passively, Aristotelian Fitlosophers are cognisant of the importance that routine and habits herald for future goals. Aristotle believes that actions counted as being "virtuous" when in alignment with an individual's human spirit—in layman's terms, their set of values—and are chosen for their own merit.

In short: a person selects an action based on their own set of values, allowing for temperance and moderation in the way they act.

Aristotle goes on to suggest that a person may lead a "good life" when they set in motion the harmony of their habits and principles of action, as this allows them to have a clear vision as to what is truly "right." Thus, an Aristotelian Fitlosopher is one who may prioritise smaller habits based on a system of values rather than focus on a specific event or goal. They will appreciate the art of moderation, knowing that both sickly indulgence or puritanical rigidity reforms of being overpowered by routines, in different extremes.

Thus, Aristotelian Fitlosophers tend to be organised and habit-based (although that's not to say outcomes aren't important) in order not to be swept away by impulse or strong emotion. They're excellent at establishing a training routine and may have a balanced, solid relationship with food or have a good grasp as to how to temper mental health woes.

So, What Exactly Is the Good Life, Then?

For Aristotle, ethical inquiry involves examining the factors required for a human to flourish based on their own nature. According to Aristotle, he defines a good life as acting in line with one's own virtues, and helping other humans lead their lives with dignity and integrity requires action and habituation. For consistency, we will revolve around this definition in this series. Excellence, therefore, must be expanded upon if we are to delve into his philosophy further.

Aristotle divides excellence in different formats:

1. Intellectual excellence: intellectual humility, logic, reasoning. May be trained by teaching others.

2. Ethical excellence: ethos, character, courage, moderation. Must be trained by habit and practice over time.

In essence, Aristotle believes that in order to *be* excellent, one must actually *practice* excellence. Therefore, if an individual is brought up practicing certain activities and associating said activities with pleasure or pain, this will reflect in their daily habits and in what they perceive to be hard. For example, if exercise has always been seen as something scary in your PE classes as a kid, or you've constantly thought you're "bad" at exercise in general, undoubtedly forming this as a habit will feel more painful than an individual who has a yogi instructor as a mum or a naturally active disposition.

Fun fact: Aristotle essentially espouses behaviourist theory, stating that children should be rewarded or punished according to their habits and desires—the BF Skinner of the ancient world.

Either of these options is no bad thing; it merely pinpoints how you may have to approach practicing leading a good life, according to Aristotle. Certain habits of yours may require more practice for them to seamlessly slot into your lifestyle.

The Aristotelian Fitlosopher

The Aristotelian Fitlosopher, therefore, has a good grasp on what habit change entails and tends to comprehend the underpinning benefits of moderation. It's not so much that they're "naturally disciplined," but much like Aristotle, they believe that in order to succeed in achieving their goals, they must continually practice certain habits in order to obtain a specific outcome.

An Aristotelian Fitlosopher might be the type of person to journal weekly habits or goals and tick off certain tasks that have been accomplished or see their overarching desire to be something that accumulates to who they want to be.

They are more likely to attribute physical prowess and achievements to accentuate certain traits or activities beyond the gym. For instance, they'll appreciate the benefits given when practicing the art of delaying gratification; they'll realise it's not merely abstaining from something but rather understanding the importance of prioritising specific actions at that moment for a greater level of overall happiness. They comprehend the difference between hedonistic fancies and longstanding contentment and are accepting of the potential tradeoff that comes with it: forgoing frequent takeaways, knowing that moderation enhances the taste in any case, for the sake of pursuing a goal larger and more purposeful than a pizza box.

If these phrases feel familiar to you, you may naturally be more inclined toward the Aristotelian way of living a fit and healthy life:

1. "I don't really like counting calories, but I do enjoy making a habit out of eating healthy and well. I have a habit tracker that helps keep me accountable."
2. "Practice makes perfect. It's about small, manageable actions that lead to the greater outcome I want."
3. "After each rep/walk/cooking session, I suck a little bit less at that activity."
4. "I like to start the day off right, with a good breakfast/bit of movement/lifting session/some meditation and journalling."

Just like Aristotle sought out the correct course of action to lead a worthy life, so too may Aristotelian Fitlosophers dictate that a certain path is a way to achieving certain goals or getting healthier. They may assume a particular way of training, or research, or even dieting is the preferred function of lifestyle change. This is exceptionally useful in carving out steely resolve and consistency, two such factors which can be lackadaisical in many individuals. They'll likely be the ones to easily eschew temptation at the dinner table when with family or friends, espousing some ethical spiel regarding habits and values and feeling better for turning down a second helping Auntie Diane's Victoria sponge.

It should be noted that whilst aware and habitual creatures, they do not deprive themselves; much like Aristotle, they value the importance of moderation. To moderate a certain amount of hedonism and pleasure as opposed to cutting it out completely is arguably more taxing on one's own will and cognition, as it requires much more pre-contemplation and awareness of one's own desires and whims. Ignoring a certain food group or social night or habit almost becomes willful ignorance rather than addressing the behaviours and thoughts and emotions that crop up when you eat a bit of chocolate cake or why you'd rather binge-watch *Tiger Hunter* instead of training after work. There's no growth, and there's no practical exertion of one's own inner strength. Aristotelian Fitlosophers are aware of this and thus are happy to have their slice of cake—they just know when it's appropriate to eat it.

The Aristotelian Fitlosopher nonetheless has to contend with the notion that their idea of the "ideal" function to health and fitness is non-linear and is quite often an intangible concept. It is natural for Aristotelian Fitlosophers to wax lyrical about the function of fitness, but why assume there is a function, and why assume there is a *unique* one? "What is *the* function of paper" (writing, wrapping, lining, etc.)? This is often a criticism Aristotelian philosophers meet when discussing virtue ethics and finding functionality in how one must lead a good life. As Robert Louden puts it, in a far more succinct way than I ever could:

> Virtues are not simply dispositions to behave in specified ways, for which rules and principles can always be cited. In addition, they involve skills of perception and articulation, situation-specific "know-how," all of which are developed only through recognizing and acting on what is relevant in concrete moral contexts as they arise. These skills of moral perception and practical reason are not completely routinizable, and so cannot be transferred from agent to agent as any sort of decision procedure... Due to the very nature of

the moral virtues, there is thus a very limited amount of advice on moral quandaries that one can reasonably expect from the virtue-oriented approach.

Here, we define the term "agent" as an ordinary, run-of-the-mill human being. If we apply this reasoning to health and fitness, we can start to see how routines are actually context-specific and require more nuance and flexibility than we can see in the rigid formats that might be espoused by Aristotelian Fitlosophers. By assuming that fitness is a monolith, Aristotelian Fitlosophers not only miss out on exciting opportunities for growth or self-development but also run the risk of ostracising methods utilised by other people.

Of course, this doesn't mean eschewing science or research in what they convey. But a prime example of this might be a strength and conditioning aficionado or a yogi keen on mobility who is "anti-aesthetics." Indeed, there is no doubt that for the former, much research demonstrates amelioration of fitness levels and muscle mass with exertion against gravity using weight, such as a barbell or dumbbell. Similarly, more and more research points to the advantage of the ground reaction being an excellent primer for fitness and getting more powerful, particularly for sports-specific tasks such as golf. This offers time-starved people a great chance at getting fit without zipping off to a gym or sacrificing time at home with the family: this type of training can be done purely based on body weight.

The aforementioned Aristotelian Fitlosopher in this hypothetical scenario, the puritan yogi, might look their nose up toward ideals that drive toward looking a certain way—and in a sense, they have a reason. There is a multitude of sociocultural drivers at bay that persuade us to pursue a path orientated around the superficial. These drivers, however, miss out on the fact that weight loss or sculpting one's own body does not, in its own standing, have to be solely a vain feat. Rather, it could represent something much more personal and powerful for an individual: losing weight to feel more energetic and being able to spend more quality time with their children, for instance.

Further to this, Aristotelian Fitlosophers advocate for moderatism and a sense of balance and refinement in their lives. As mentioned, this is an excellent way to practice a diligent attitude toward one's own goals and letting the benefits of routine and exercising self-control bleed out into the rest of their lives. Nonetheless, when it comes to general athleticism, and even life itself, there will be times when something more stringent, perhaps gregarious or even extreme, may be called for.

Take, for instance, the average martial artist or successful fighter. For them, taking on a hobbyist approach to the sport they partake in would be a recipe for disaster and loss. In order to reach the highest level, and thus their goal, they must be willing to sacrifice, at the very least, temporarily, certain pleasures and habits that have allowed them the luxury of moderation. They must push themselves beyond the remit of performing a task for wellbeing or self-development. For them, it becomes something more. A chance to truly advance in both body and mind.

I am certainly not suggesting people quit their day jobs and try to become the next UFC star. But evidently, there is some merit for choosing to invest extra time and dedication into a certain facet of one's life, at least at various, temporary points during a lifetime. Knowing that you can reach beyond preconceived limits set by your mind or societal mores and push yourself past the ordinary, everyday rhythm of routine is enormously empowering. Moderation and temperament are absolutely things to strive for, at least 90 percent of the time—but Aristotelian Fitlosophers may miss out on the thrill, excitement, and, more importantly, exponential growth in character that comes with pushing oneself past moderation for a greater goal than themselves.

How can an Aristotelian Fitlosopher learn to find fluidity in their views?

It's important to realise that if you do fall on the side of Aristotelian Fitlosophy, then odds are, you have cultivated a strong habitual base and are able to pull off routine and goal-based activities with aplomb. There's also a very strong chance that you exert a flexible kind of thinking and are able to be open-minded toward different approaches, including ones that err toward immoderate stints to achieve a greater goal. Oddly enough, it's likely you'll have an argument for these kinds of models in a way that is solidly Aristotelian.

Like with any approach, there runs the risk of taking it too far, and so if you've found yourself becoming too rigid or inappropriately stalwart to your own routine, it might be worth being able to adopt that flexible, open-ended thinking that we discussed previously.

This is where we can adapt to being slightly more superfluous, slightly more open-ended than the methodical journey of Aristotle's logic-based rhetoric. Rather than thinking about going from A to B to C, we can consider an array of other variations by considering our own **personal constructs** toward a situation. Here, a theory was proposed by clinician George Kelly. This theory may very well suit an individual more attuned to Aristotelian logic, as the concept is orientated around human beings trying to understand each other and navigate the world around them.

Kelly, similar to Aristotle's notion of logic, believed that we try to come up with hypotheses and attempt to prove or disprove them as life progresses. In a sense, he suggests we are something like scientists of life, and we create our own personal constructs used to perceive and interpret events. We then act according to said perception. Where Kelly's approach differs from an Aristotelian approach, however, lies in the outcome of this construct. We are free to be creative in how we perceive and how we evaluate what constructs may benefit.

This concept allows us to examine the events in our lives a bit more flexibly. Rather than adhere to a strict cause-and-effect sort of thinking, we are able to be slightly future-orientated in how we act and the way we format goals. With Aristotelian logic, there may be a tendency, if not careful, to ignore the outcome and look at the validity of the path at hand. In terms of how we manifest that into the realm of fitness and health, for instance, one might become fixated on a certain habit or activity to feel "safe" or solidify their constructed logic of a certain approach. This is something I like to refer to as **Utility Belt Syndrome**; a fervent need or desire to engage in a certain habit or wear a specific type of trainer or eat your favourite breakfast, lest the day stops in its tracks.

How Can I Be Less Aristotle, More Full-Throttle?

We can prevent this by channeling the way we process a task or event at hand into how we anticipate events by developing and capitalising on our need to explore both inner and outer worlds. We may construe our environments via our personal construct, rather than the other way round, and navigate ourselves in this unpredictable world according to both short-term and future goals. As a result, we are staunch on the outcome but flexible regarding the path we take to get there.

Flexible thinking can be a challenge, particularly when we live in a time whereby certainty and loud claims make for popularity. It can be exceptionally challenging to think about different ways to . . . well, think. Some of the following can help trigger that cognitive flexibility, particularly if you feel a bit stuck in a psychological rut:

1. Pick up a new hobby that gets you really excited, regardless of its perceived "value" in terms of formalised goals or profession.
2. Question your own thoughts and thinking, and observe the language you use about certain topics or in conversation generally.
3. Change up your regular routine in a way that does not feel too perturbing. For example, your evening/morning walk could be altered in its route somewhat to create a modicum of spontaneity.
4. Expose yourself to a variety of beliefs, morality systems, values, and expectations—particularly in regards to the different ways people stay fit and healthy.

It's vital to remember this: that the Aristotelian Fitlosopher is likely to already have a solid grasp on cultivating habits and achieving their goals. It comes naturally for them, as it aligns with their values of practicing virtue, and as a result developing excellence for themselves and in their eyes for others. This is not to say this base logic is inherently invalid, unsound, or a hindrance in itself. This section merely serves as a reminder for those who err toward this tendency that there is value in "bending the rules," so to speak, and being able to either fully relax or indulge at times or even push themselves beyond a preconceived boundary.

Aristotle was a philosopher preoccupied with substance, which he categorised into form and matter. Form was used to categorise what kind of thing the object was, and matter is used to describe precisely what this is made of. We can use his logic as a result without veering off into subjective or constructivist arguments. Aristotle viewed substances as being those things on which the existence of everything else depends and on which our systematic knowledge depends. We can thus tailor our view of lifestyle and fitness according to this premise, without compromising our ways of thinking or logical functions.

By tweaking these contingencies, it becomes less inexorable to alter the way we view lifestyle change. Sometimes that discomfort we experience forms a **cognitive dissonance**, and it feels as though any other point of view or contribution, try as hard as we might, simply doesn't fit into what we perceive to be "true." Sometimes by reframing an argument into one that suits our own worldview or logical machinations, it becomes an easier pill to swallow: that just because the end goal may be the same doesn't mean you aren't able to manifest that result through different paths.

SOCRATES AND THE SOCRATIC FITLOSOPHER

Socrates, arguably one of the most influential thinkers in ancient and modern philosophy, was quite a controversial figure, so much so that he was regularly mocked in the various plays shown by Athenians and sentenced to death for "corrupting the youth" of Athens. That's what you get for encouraging people to think for themselves, apparently. Even though we still have so much to unearth about this enigmatic philosopher, his death has become a longstanding symbol for the concept of philosophy.

In a nutshell: he remains a relative mystery even in contemporary terms, as shockingly, he has written nothing down. All of our hypotheses and theories surrounding his ideas and theories stem from second-hand assertions from his followers and are hotly debated. This difficulty in discerning fact from myth has been dubbed as the Socratic problem, and as a result, what academics have concluded is that we do not necessarily have a grasp on who the real Socrates is, but merely theories and postulations and scatterings of ideas on a man, or motif, who has single-handedly created a symbol for philosophers everywhere.

Consequently, trying to decide exactly what Socrates thought and how he presented it becomes a bit muddled; we end up having to rely on secondary accounts and theories, even by various propositions today that have little to no link with ancient times. For the sake of consistency, in this part of the series, we'll be making assumptions based on the recorded conversations with his followers, like Plato and Xenophon.

Similar to the way Aristotle viewed philosophy, Socrates believed that philosophy should be at its heart practical for the good of society and involved itself not in conveying knowledge but rather asking question after clarifying question until his students arrived at their own understanding. We dub this theory the **Socratic Method**. Much of his stuff has actually percolated into modern-day psychotherapeutic treatment today—the benefit/cost analysis we saw earlier in this series, for instance—as well as political democracy at large.

Funnily enough, Socrates is one of the fair few philosophers who opine directly on the concept of exercise and fitness, using the basis of these underpinning ethics. He noted that those who were well-trained were physically primed to go to war, honour their friends, and improve their own mood. He adds, in that paraphrased, oft-quoted citation, that it becomes a shame for an individual to pass by life and not see the person they can become. For Socrates, exercise was a vessel to become a better person.

Socratic Fitlosophers will probably share this view, concluding that their need to train isn't based on a superficial desire but one of personal development. Socratic Fitlosophers may believe that the need to train carries a deeper drive to help others, knowing that they cannot fill others' cups if their own is empty. This may lead to greater conscientiousness or discipline.

Known for his debate skills, Socrates was adept at sniffing out logical fallacies and underlying biases in an argument. This has become a well-known trope among schools and thoughts in philosophy too. A Socratic Fitlosopher may therefore be well-adjusted to applying this same skepticism and logic toward fitness myths. They'll likely be the first to question their own biases whilst also annoying the living crap out of people (just like Socrates did) by thought-vomiting onto others and goading them for discussion or debate. Obviously, they might do well by learning to quiet their mind from time to time and being open to lighten themselves up rather than buckling down if they become overly neurotic.

According to the Socratic Method, a statement may be considered true only if it cannot be proved wrong. This methodology breaks down a problem into a series of questions, with the aim that these are then sought to be answered. This method, now also used in scientific research by making a hypothesis and then either proving it correct or false, can be infuriating if done right. Socrates was famous for outlining the flaws and follies of his intellectual opponents by asking what appear to be, on the surface, highly innocent questions.

The Socratic Method is an excellent toe-dip into the world of philosophical arguments and critical thinking. Regardless if you click with this way of thinking when it comes to daily life, it's still worth considering his approach, even if you tend to think about these kinds of things differently.

That's All Very Well and Good—But How Can Being an Insufferable Know-It-All Help Me Get Fitter?

A Socratic Fitlosopher may have the gift of critical thinking, being able to sniff out an incoherent argument a mile away and address it accordingly. One glance at the 'Gram, for instance, simply cements this as being a highly versatile skill to wield indeed. Knowing the difference between shiny photos or videos and a decent following versus a genuine, profound knowledge and respect for research will take one very far in their own goals—and life in general.

What's more, there is always one universal from the Socratic Method that I take away and apply to my clients: getting to the bottom of their approach, their goals, and their values by asking question after question, in typical Socratic style, in order to ascertain the background behind why they came to me.

	Why?	Why?
So?		
So?		

The Why-Why/So-So dialogue is a very interesting concept that mirrors the way Socrates would try and dissect an illogical argument. Not to say that a client's goals or the way you want to get from A to B is illogical—we just want to try and cement a purpose into the reason why you're trying to get to a certain destination. We want to assure ourselves that there is a deeper resonance, an intense yearning, and hunger, to better ourselves, and by proxy, add to the world around us.

The Socratic Fitlosopher

Why-Why/So-So is a standard method of procedure for the Socratic Fitlosopher. They tend to want to know that their deadlifts serve a greater purpose than just picking up something heavy and putting it back down again and dig into the trenches of their psyche to find out what may work for them and their worldview and what may not.

A client, for instance, may demand that they want to lose weight or get fitter simply because. Or that they don't feel comfortable in their own skin. Or that they could stand to lose a few pounds, and then they'd feel a little bit better.

This is all very well and good for a generalised outline of a goal in general, but as a coach, my personal philosophy (heh) would be to try and find the root cause of this desire.

Desire	Why?	So?
I want to lose weight to look/ feel a bit better.	I feel self-conscious around my friends.	So, losing weight would help my sense of self and help me feel more like I fit in.

An example of how one could delve into the reasoning behind their own drive and goals.

Upon probing, Sarah might suggest that her insecurities lie not in the weight loss itself but in the mere notion that she doesn't quite feel as happy as she could be with her group of friends and peers. As we know, humans are social creatures; Socrates would explore this phenomenon further, suggesting Sarah's degree of feeling this rejection may infiltrate into daily life and how she interacts with others. She may become more surly, cynical, or anxious and thus be lacking in her overall contributions to societal or practical well-being.

The weight loss goal, therefore, becomes something much more than merely aesthetic or surface-level. A Socratic Fitlosopher will eviscerate, explore, and excavate reasons and musings behind their goals in order to feel purposeful and meaningful in how they train and eat. There will always need to be a what, why, and so in order for them to fully comprehend the process and follow through with it.

If you err on the trend of Socratic Fitlosopher, you might find yourself uttering the following:

1. *An example of how one could delve into the reasoning behind their own drive and goals.* "For me, if I exercise, I feel better. If I feel better, I can be a better friend/partner/sibling/child."
2. *An example of how one could delve into the reasoning behind their own drive and goals.* "But isn't it true if something claims to fix posture, and makes someone 'feel better,' then that is merely correlative, and instead they've helped to soothe the nervous system and thus aid in them feeling confident physically and mentally?"
3. "I always feel sluggish if I eat lots of junk or don't move much. I feel like I can't focus or I'm grumpy with everyone."
4. "Knowing that ticking off this activity or cooking this meal might help set me up to do good for others genuinely excites me."

For a Socratic Fitlosopher, it may be inexorably difficult to get started on a regime unless they have their own guiding star, whispering sweet everything into their ear and assuring them that what they do has purpose and meaning.

Like the Aristotelian Fitlosopher, this premise is one that appears to be a pretty solid way to build one's foundation of values and goal-orientated behaviour. There runs a risk, moreover, of being almost too fixed and too rigid with the way we view our world and, by proxy, ourselves.

Picture the scene. Imagine you are at a dinner party, a reunion evening, the room filled with various characters and the hum of warm chatter and excitement and clattering of knives and forks. All these people are wonderfully unique, carrying different values and experiences and worldly views, nattering away and discussing the current shitshow that is contemporary culture.

There's a minor caveat to this metaphor. All of these people, in their wonderful differences and uniqueness, are you. They are Past You, Potential You, You from childhood who never quite outgrew their obsession for Pokémon or anime (just ask Present You.) And all these Yous carry with them past actions, values, and regrets which differ from You to You.

Going to chat with Childhood You might see their values system align with becoming a marine biologist or riding the biggest rollercoaster in Disneyland Paris. Teenage You might see a values system of getting into the best university or dating the best-looking person at school. Early-Twenties You might be a bit more solid, looking toward important goals and markers of purpose such as finding a fulfilling career or learning to communicate better in relationships. As each You ages, you'll find these values and arbiters of meaning differ. They may become more solid and less conceptual, chasing after not an intangible dream but something that can be easily digestible and achieved by actions and habits.

Between these values lie the rust-caked remnants of past regret and lingering pain. It's the embarrassing, clumsy actions of a pained ex or the overtly emotional outburst of younger selves past when coming across failure.

Your actual self has two options here: to understand and learn and forgive that past You for doing the best that they could, comprehending their actions, and seeing how far their values have come in the long run. Option two is to psychologically punish your former present. The dinner party is abruptly ruined; Future-Career You's eyes widen at the sight of you downing your fifth tequila shot, blustering unintelligible insults drenched in shame. "Why were you such a dumbass? Can't you do anything right? Why do you fuck up all the time?"

The rest of the guests shift in their seats, a visceral tension biting through the air. Who invited this Me, they may wonder. Future-Career You nods sagely, reminiscing the times that Present You lambasted themselves with shame and self-loathing and hurtful actions.

This long-winded metaphor has a point, I promise.

Our present actions motivated by our cornerstone principles are representative of our current, higher-level values that guide us and set the scene for how we behave and navigate the world around us. Ultimately, how we view our actions and the way we interpret our actions allows us to create higher-level forms of purpose and permits us to grow and be fully functioning adults, rather than aimlessly wandering adolescents wearing fancy suits.

Thankfully, our values are not as fixed or as cemented as we may first presume. Anytime we are faced with a life crisis or meet with a mentor, or therapist, or confidant in general, we are given the opportunity to analyse the way we interpret our actions and carry out those daily actions according to what we value.

Socrates advocated for leading a certain lifestyle as a kind of transcended means to an end. To exercise is not merely making yourself healthy or fit but instead to become a better person overall, and by proxy, become a better human being for society and contribute unconditionally.

Naturally, a Socratic Fitlosopher will stick to these guns, arguably to the point whereby they almost gnaw their own fingers off in inundated neuroticism, and chastise their former selves for being so immature, so vulgar, so out of line with the values they espouse *now*.

The fact is, regret is no picnic, but that doesn't mean that it's inherently bad or wrong, either. We require this byproduct of evolutionary processing in order to continually evaluate and adjust our behaviours and actions or be cast out by society and condemned to a lonely, isolated life. If we *didn't* feel bad or embarrassed about past behaviours or ideas, then that would be more worrying. We would be stuck in a fixed mindset as opposed to a growth one, never acknowledging when we fucked up or when it might be appropriate to change a mindset for the sake of others around us and ourselves.

Self-loathing, on the other hand, can be the next level down from shame and regret. Self-loathing paralyses us, preventing action and learning from occurring as we continually play whack-a-mole with every gnawing, excruciating pang of pain that crops up, eventually beating ourselves to a pulp. Self-loathing is childishly extreme, forgetting where we were at that time and that we had all the skills at our disposal then and were simply doing our best at the time. Self-loathing decontextualises any other factors that may have contributed to our behaviours, such as external stress, past trauma, and problematic interpersonal relationships, thus shifting all the blame onto ourselves as opposed to simply taking responsibility and owning our flaws. Self-loathing can quickly descend into self-pity, making it almost impossible to communicate your fears to another without frustrating the living hell out of them.

Take it from somebody who still struggles with the seductive whispers of giving in and believing that failure and misery is the only route: self-loathing can be as corrosive as hubristic arrogance, and in its own sense, has its own air of doleful narcissism permeating its core. After all, you're not that special to warrant being the only person in the universe never to experience pain or never face setbacks. One of the beautiful things about being human is that: we are all messy, flawed, perhaps a bit broken, and paradoxically it is in that acceptance that we are able to examine the values guiding us and act accordingly.

I truly believe that there is a pitfall in becoming too urgent, too fixated in the way we perceive self-development and personal change. There's a chance that those who err on the side of the Socratic Fitlosopher may indeed fall trap to this way of thinking, too. What was once an impetus for growth and responsibility now becomes something quite stultifying, suffocating your choices and worldview as you spiral into a descent of self-loathing and refusal for acceptance. And when you struggle to accept yourself, you vie for others to do the accepting for you. You meekly hunt for validation, consciously or unconsciously, unable to sate the entrenched abyss seeping beyond your insides. An incessant search for change, or a belief that you *have* to change in order to be a valid human being, is not the same as thorough self-responsibility and eschewing pleasure over true happiness.

Wow, that got dark *quick*.

Having values and knowing that a certain activity transcends its material conditions is an excellent attribute, and Socratic Fitlosophers tend to be excellent at putting off momentary pleasure for longer-lasting contentment and a sense of well-being. Further, their critical thinking skills are probably second to none; they question age-old aphorisms in the industry, are unafraid to ponder upon notions that don't quite sit well with them, and are happy to sift through the research if needed.

But the constant chase for change and self-improvement can prove to be mentally exhausting and, in the end, self-defeating. The very thing we try to avoid becomes our fate in the end due to burnout and a generally unstable sense of self. There are better ways of being able to stick to a lifestyle routine without chipping away at your own being.

What's the Right Balance Between the Socratic Method and Annoying the Living Hell Out of People?

Socratic Fitlosophers might do well to take a step back and—bear with me for a sec—use their brains less.

They'll naturally be more inclined to analytical thinking and questioning themselves to the nth degree, to the point whereby they'll be living a routine of rigidity and stiffness to fulfill the perceived fulfillment that their values give them.

Humans are creatures bound by both genetic and neurobiological components in addition to their experiential and sociological surroundings. We often discuss the benefits of psychological grit and emotional resilience, espoused by thinkers such as the Stoics and Socrates himself. Without dismissing the importance of this development, a hyper-focus on the individual and a stern grasp on our own loci of control may fail to capture the complex, fluctuating, unpredictable forces that are more readily apparent when we try, fail, and try again to navigate the maelstrom of our own society.

Psychological flexibility has been a concept promoted by several theories, including Acceptance and Compassion Therapy and other offshoots of CBT. Rather than attempting to recreate my own half-baked explanation, I'll leave it to Kashdan and Rottenburg—from the pair's review paper, "Psychological Flexibility as a Fundamental Aspect of Health," published in Volume 30, Issue 4 of *Clinical Psychology Review* in 2010—to do the work for me:

> Recognize and adapt to various situational demands; shift mindsets or behavioral repertoires when these strategies compromise personal or social functioning; maintain balance among important life domains; and be aware, open, and committed to behaviors that are congruent with deeply held values.

Whilst it can be difficult to view health in terms of defined schemas and markers we can identify boundaries of objectivity on a spectrum, at least. Psychopathology on average presents itself when this inability to adapt to these circumstantial demands becomes a frequent issue for an individual. A depressive episode becomes something that interferes with human function and fundamental needs, for instance, when somebody refuses to get out of bed all day or self-harms. This rigidity of how they view themselves in addition to the world around them is paralysing.

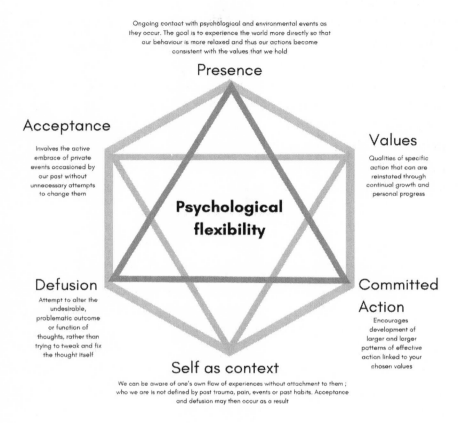

A visual example of the ACT (Acceptance and Compassion-based Therapy) "Hexaflex" model, originally designed by Steven C. Hayes and recreated here by Sophie Thomas.

This is not a hyperbolic point of contention to argue that Socratic Fitlosophers are on the same level as an individual with depression or as someone who struggles with emotional repression. I'd even argue that their ability to critique and analyse may also act as a great weapon against some forms of automatic, irrational thoughts.

But it's worth acknowledging that purpose, meaning, and values aren't necessarily set in stone. Psychological flexibility may be pertinent for a Socratic Fitlosopher if they find themselves becoming an overt slave to routine and attitudes. Tapping into that sweet spot of uncovering different ways to skin a cat, so to speak, will not only allow for more open-mindedness in your own journey but enable better conversations and understanding of the paths other people choose to undertake.

NIETZSCHE AND THE NIETZSCHEAN FITLOSOPHER

Alongside Kant, Friedrich Nietzsche (1844–1900) is undoubtedly the most famous (and perhaps most memes) philosopher spoken about in contemporary discussion. His writings spanned a wide array of topics, including the origins of truth, history, power, morality, nihilism, and the meaning of existence. He was quite the philosophical polymath, as can be assumed. His writings have exerted an enormous influence on Western philosophy and intellectual history, and a fair few of the ideas he conceived are easily palatable in YouTube videos or discourse on self-development.

Understandably, to even scratch the surface of what Nietzsche intended to evoke in his philosophy would require a dissertation at a minimum and a multitude of books for the best levels of depth, such things that we do not have here at our disposal. We do, however, have several parallels running through his writings and how we apply these lessons in a practical setting—or, moreover, when we set goals to get fitter and healthier. A bit like the stoics, some of Nietzsche's ideas have turned out rather nicely in terms of pragmatism and utility, and many of us utter the odd aphorism and live by certain aligned values that, incidentally, live up to Nietzschean principles.

It's apt to discuss one of Nietzsche's most-famed of lines, "God is dead. God remains dead. And we have killed him." This parable was uttered initially in his work *The Gay Science* but became a striking theme and feature of one of his more popular works, *Thus Spoke Zarathustra*. Much contentious debate surrounds it; some argue that Nietzsche embraces a kind of nihilism, rejecting metaphysical and religious claims in favour of exploring the human conditions in more poetic terms, denying conventional forms of "truth" or "knowledge." However, a more popular reading of this phrase is one that engages in reaffirming life through a constant, radical reprogramming of human existence, morality, and knowledge. Whichever route you take, the general premise of Nietzsche is thus: for Nietzsche, developing meaning in life is a plan that requires constant struggle with one's psychological and intellectual inheritances.

Nietzsche discusses the literal human metamorphoses in his masterpiece Thus Spake Zarathustra. This work is highly Campbellian in nature—even when conveyed in a stern, bold tone, the outline of *The Hero's Journey* is plain for all to see in his writing. The work is a metaphor for human evolution, representing the paradigm shift we must face in certain stages of our life. In Nietzsche's eyes, we may start out as sheep—meek, and part of the herd, following what is societally expected of us. It is in Nietzsche's hopes that we percolate from sheep to camel, all the way to lion. The lion realises it is futile to fight against anything and everything, and the final and most important stage is the transformation from lion to child. The child has the opportunity, now, to carry out their own meaning and live for living's sake, adopting curiosity and resilience as opposed to a fruitless resistance against life's maelstrom.

Nietzsche is often cited amidst self-developmental literature, alongside purveyors and practitioners of the stoic philosophy. Contrary to condemnatory reviews and superficial readings, Nietzsche was probably the most anti-German nationalist and humane thinker you could find. His sister, a known member of a far-right party and fervent anti-Semite, utilised his work after his death and propagated them via mistranslations and poor publications to be politically driven. As you can imagine, in reality, Nietzsche was especially apolitical given his skepticism on its effect on the human condition. Accusations of anti-Semitism in his work are unfounded.

As such, Nietzsche asserted that a truly noble, exemplary human being would be one to eschew transcendent coping mechanisms— the arts, poetry, religion, or the notion of a soul—in doing so, craft out their own identity and values beyond those lying within society's grasp. Nietzsche was very well known for his rebellious attitude, both in his personal affairs and philosophical outlook. It comes as no surprise that his ideas have stood the test of time in terms of popularity. He also makes for an intriguing and compelling template in our Fitlosophy series, particularly when we think about overcoming conventional aphorisms to encourage personal authenticity.

All Work and No Play...?

The Gay Science is one of Nietzsche's most beautiful and important books. Yet it was never received with lauding or appraisal; only one meagrely translated edition was published in the twilight days of post–World War I. Indeed, Nietzsche was seen as a heretic or a madman for the majority of his life. Teased for his total lack of gentlemanly charm and furtive appearance, his writings, bold and exclamatory and exhilarating, appear a far cry from the sullen slip of a man portrayed in journals and biographical records.

As any good philosopher with a sense of humour does, Nietzsche tells the reader that "this entire book is really nothing but an amusement." Naturally, one must keep in mind that a philosopher's amusement (and especially Nietzsche's amusement) may bear little resemblance to that of the average person. But can a philosopher's amusement still be something philosophical? Or is anything lighthearted and gay necessarily frivolous—a mere diversion from the serious business of pursuing the truth? These questions lie at the heart of *The Gay Science.*

Nietzsche explored these themes in conjunction with confronting the lack of meaning present in society. Though he didn't quite live long enough to ascertain what that transformative element would be, he did pinpoint some key trends we are seeing emerge as of late:

1. The attenuation of influences like writing, art, and religion would lead people to try and find meaning in extreme political alignments or socially materialist movements.
2. He believed that an increase in daily comforts would lead to an accumulation of nihilism and existential dread.

"Thus Spoke Online Fitness Classes...?"

A Nietzschean Fitlosopher, with this in mind, might be the kind of person to face challenge square in the eye and laugh at its inane attempts to disparage or disarm. They are much more likely to accept that changing one's dietary, fitness, and overall lifestyle habits is not a linear concept, and as such, have a higher chance of putting themselves out there in competitions or events, choosing adversity as the method to better themselves. Instead of shying away from a challenge, they embrace it. A Stoic Fitlosopher is accepting no matter what the outcome; a Nietzschean Fitlosopher, on the other hand, is more likely to go out there and actively seek out hardship. Think of a bodybuilding competition, martial arts competition, or even a running challenge.

Given Nietzsche's disdain toward comforts and idyllic ways of living, it makes sense that a Nietzschean Fitlosopher would follow suit and reject notions of rest and comfort in order to grow, physically or mentally.

You might be more inclined toward Nietzschean values if the following phrases seem in keeping with your personality and habits:

- "The only way I can get better or push myself is doing something I might not enjoy at that moment, but I know it's good for me."
- "I've just entered this fight/comp/marathon/event. Let's see how I'll learn and grow from this."
- "Life's not worth living without some challenge or stress to overcome."
- "I might be limited with equipment/finances/access to knowledge, but damnit, am I gonna do what I can with what I have."

Nietzschean Fitlosophers may generally be associated with that rough-and-tumble attitude of getting tough as the tough gets going, so to speak. Naturally, they form admirable value pillars and ways of navigating themselves through stressful periods, maintaining routine even when they feel burdened; their resilience levels are higher as a result.

Nietzsche was a philosopher, moreover, who argued that our intentions were bookended by self-centred desires. This is not analogous to saying that individuals are selfish, reprehensible figures; it's a complicated layering of how we interpret good deeds. For instance, a well-renowned doctor might be apt in treating their patients and claim that they may take on the most challenging of cases purely to help them get better. But Nietzsche would argue that, deep down, this doctor might seek out such medical conundrums not necessarily to chase after altruism but to better himself and carve out value as a doctor. Inevitably, said patients would go away and gush their praises across the town about this professional's craft, elevating the doctor in both integrity and status.

This is not to say that all good deeds are forms of manipulation per se, but Nietzsche prods at us to embrace ourselves before yoking others into accepting or liking us. In short, Nietzsche considered the act of people-pleasing or acting to please others a mewling, emasculating approach. Rather, he posited the need for us to live authentically, whether or not people like or do not like who we are. What matters most is how we design ourselves and whether or not what we do and how we live are in accordance with our deepest values. How many times, after all, do you feel compelled to approach that one person at the party who has that intangible, *je ne sais quo aura* surrounding their personhood? How many times do you think, *God, they're pretty cool* as you saunter past them, recalling another scandalous anecdote, footsteps as light as pebbles as you furtively yearn for mutual eye contact? And yet, what makes this aura all the more palpable is the simple, undeniable fact that this individual likely doesn't give a shit about what you think about them.

A Nietzschean Fitlosopher, simply put, understands that following another path for the sake of familiarity or tradition is a setup for sheer, bone-aching misery. One diet might ensure a brighter, more self-assured disposition for one person but an ache of dissatisfaction in another. More broadly, a Nietzschean Fitlosopher recognises the futility of following another's predilections and preferences. Nietzsche would likely question whether this individual was really living at all—a puff of vapid, lukewarm existence rather than truly embracing what life offers us.

An example of someone not abiding by this sense of authenticity would be a fitness influencer on social media touting the latest GymShark leggings or tea cleanse. In this instance, this individual is part of the groupthink; there is no querying the status quo, no elevated cognition beyond that of a consumer mentality. There's nothing particularly wrong about choosing this line of fitness and well-being (though one may very well make the robust, moral argument as to why they shouldn't espouse faddish diet trends), but it implies a diluted sense of self. Whilst Nietzsche's own self-elected loneliness should be taken with a handful of salt; he made great strides to avoid the influence of generic opening and the more "obvious" paths in life. A Nietzschean Fitlosopher might abscond from the typical "bro" gym buff image that pervades society, Tom Ford cologne and all, but finds deeper meaning going for a solo stroll, golf club in tow, or eating pizza without posting it compulsively on Instagram to assure others of alleged spontaneity. Hashtag goals.

Finding Your Nietzsche in the Market

A Nietzschean Fitlosopher is all about carving out their own individual path, preferences, and purpose in the hunt for the holy grail of health.

But is there such a thing as being too individualistic in the pursuit of one's own goals? I speak of this problem again when referring to the Objectivist school of thought (see Chapter 5). Treading your own journey, according to Nietzsche, is a noble form of authenticity. One eschews pleasing others and refuses to be held captive by societal "niceties"; they march to the beat of their own drum, you could say. A Nietzschean Fitlosopher might be so hellbent on following their own path that others' worldviews and values become a distant speck on the horizon.

Seeing conventional values or approaches to well-being as "above you," for instance, fosters a reeking, lingering air of arrogance that is harder to scrub off than red wine on a pearl-white carpet.

Ironically, seeing yourself as more "individual" and "unique" lands you in the same problem as you found yourself before; chained and entrapped by this notion, you now have to live up to the idea of being "free" or "special." In a grandiose show of intellectual snake-eating, you become the very thing you swore not to transform into.

If you, for instance, see calorie-counting or tracking your steps akin to something that only a "basic bitch" might align themselves with, then I've got some bad news: you're that person too. Finding your own values or path isn't about doing the most esoteric, quirky, potentially impractical thing you can find on this planet. Otherwise, you end up entangled in the intersect of açai brunches, jiu-jitsu cultists, and Clapham inhabitants. As someone who has, at some point in her life, slot into all three categories, I can confirm that this does not make you a special individual.

Finding your values should be something intertwined with your own authenticity, after all. Nietzsche admonishes us for following societal norms, yet we cannot deny that rejection and disconnection affect similar regions of the brain in a manner parable to that of physical pain. It goes against the evolutionary instinct to thrive in a community and be "accepted" as part of a greater whole than us. That's not to say Nietzsche is wrong in advising us to live an authentic life of our own accord, naturally. But much of what he has to say gets misinterpreted and twisted to mean, essentially "fuck everybody else," or assume traditional values like family, community, and responsibility anchor us in one spot, chain and ball and all. In actuality, one person's freedom and joy can easily be derived from such values. And another person, in equal measures, finds their own sense of self being individuated by travel, freedom, honesty, and creativity. Others, a real mix. In short, the point of Nietzsche's philosophy is to uncover what liberty looks like for you and you alone—and not let outside opinions sway you to a different way of living.

Alone, Together?

It's tempting for Nietzschean Fitlosophers to forgo the clumsy machinations teamwork can lug around with it and take off, establishing goals and pathways solely of their own volition and desires. This is not the same thing as describing their individuality as selfishness or arrogance. Certainly, it takes a degree of self-involvement to thrive in sports like bodybuilding or taking your chosen sport to an athletic degree. Deriving a sense of empowerment from eschewing social recommendations can be thrilling but at times isolating.

Not allowing your own sense of self-worth to be at the mercy of others' gossip or empty validation is a tremendous lesson we can all take from the Nietzschean Fitlosopher. Nonetheless, there is such thing as being too autonomous. To outright ignore the meaning that cooperation and active listening brings to the table results in overlooking years of literature pinpointing the importance of an other-based approach in daily life. Extroversion has been associated with higher levels of wellbeing and better quality of living, possibly due to the fact that individuals who consider themselves to be extroverts are more likely to connect with others, even strangers like the local bus driver or barista, on a regular basis. Extensive research exists on the balmy, palliative effect of social connection on the human nervous system. Safe interpersonal relationships are also strongly correlated with "correcting" prediction errors the brain makes: a highly neurotic individual's worldview that people are dangerous requires regular, comforting correspondence with others if they are able to adjust this maladaptive coping mechanism.

It might benefit the Nietzschean Fitlosopher to consider a more lenient, pliable view of lifestyle if they feel themselves becoming as sullen or outcasted as the eponymous thinker himself. A

Postmodernist approach, despite being at loggerheads with Nietzschean values of truth, offers openness and a wide array of options to assuage potential guilt, pricking at the hearts of a driven individual, reminding them that not only is it more than okay to seek company or even help, but it might even be good for their health.

AYN RAND AND THE OBJECTIVIST FITLOSOPHER

Okay, dear reader. It's here. The section I've been least looking forward to writing about the most.

Not because of this thinker's belief system, per se. But rather, the general aura of disdain I feel that some may harbour toward this philosopher, not necessarily for illogical or emotionally charged reasons.

Ayn Rand (1905–1982) is a funny one and potentially one of the heavy-hitters on this list—inevitably due to her carrying a fair deal of controversy alongside an intellectual legacy. Hell, many contemporary thinkers question whether or not she should even be considered philosophy in her totality. She focused mostly on novels, short stories, and other variants of fiction during her early career before expanding upon these works and fully outlining her comprehensive philosophical ideas. In this sense, it can be hard to, quite literally, discern fact (or premise) from fiction in many cases with her writing.

It should be stressed, as with all other thinkers in this series, that just because you may align with philosophy in terms of lifestyle and habits does not equate to your moral standpoints matching as well. In short, the truth might be this: you may see yourself more as an

Objectivist *Fitlosopher*, but beyond the scope of self-improvement or getting fitter, you belong in the left-leaning political camp or prefer virtue ethics over Rand's Darwinian view of morality.

Rand was preoccupied with the idea of attaining a kind of human perfection, and it was through philosophy that she endeavoured to seek this. One of the reasons for the skepticism toward Rand's ideas is that she essentially views laissez-faire capitalism as a means to this end; in her non-fiction works like *Atlas Shrugged* and *The Fountainhead*, she explores concepts such as "ethical egoism." In her works, Rand espouses that an individual's happiness and productivity act as the moral purposes that drive their lives. Indeed, Rand sees morality as a necessity for human beings to survive. Many philosophers talk about the notion of a "social contract," which is essentially a morality model describing the ways in which people behave and act within the confines of agreed-upon, inherent guidelines. Some people consider the relationship between government and citizens to be a type of social contract, for instance. For Rand, morality can be extracted from this social contract; in other words, for Rand, morality is a purely mechanistic feature for humans to live. Think of the scorned lover who hereby proclaims love to be a purely biological impulse to procreate, and you have a similar vein of thinking.

For Rand, the need for morality is predicated upon the fact that survival is interpolated into our veins, and so morality is needed in any situation—but not for the same reasons somebody like Kant might argue, for instance. Unlike Kant, who bases his notion of morality on duty-based behaviours (deontology, as we know it to be), there is no ethical or moral imperative to survive; if you choose to live, then you must value your own survival as part of a species as the ultimate end; morality, therefore, becomes the necessary means to achieving it. (I talk more about means and ends in the section on Kantian ethics.)

In layman's terms, your own "survival" is not merely a literal concept; it can also be described as a kind of self-responsibility for your own happiness and thriving as a human being. This is why many Republicans and right-wing figures often align their views with Rand's ideology. Self-responsibility is a notion, on average, associated with both conservative and libertarian ideas, the fact that no conglomerate or group should or can be responsible for the path you set yourself in life. Naturally, this does not have to translate to any political alignment; someone very left-wing can ascribe a high value to self-responsibility whilst believing in the power of the social collective, for instance. Nonetheless, it's the trope we still see today, littered across political billboards and loosely written manifestos.

So an Objectivist, or Randian Fitlosopher, does not have to be a worshipper of the capitalistic free market to value the importance of self-responsibility in their own lifestyle undertaking. A Randian Fitlosopher could see every action toward their goals as something that they and they alone are culpable for; the 5:00 a.m. runs, the lunchtime gym sessions, squeezed into a day of chaos and stress, and eschewing gooey chocolatey goodness each time a colleague's birthday comes into play.

Rand's view of self-ownership is dubbed by many as a form of radical responsibility. The phrase can seem somewhat off-put-ting—"radical" responsibility implies some form of extremist ad-herence to one's own life path, when, in reality, responsibility is as much a holistic action as it is a descriptive noun—but there is truth in what it sows. An Objectivist Fitlosopher, in this vein of think-ing, would typically reject envy and self-pity, instead opting for an emphasis on achievement. They are fully aware that to live by their effort guarantees a set result; conversely, they will not receive undeserved efforts if the warranted work fails to be put into play.

Isn't this the kind of stuff you see plastered by motivational quotes all over social media?

Sorta. For one, despite my disdain for Rand, I will give her credit in that, at the very least, she tries a bit harder than the average social media mogul in engaging her readers. Objectivism posits happiness as a noble moral goal. In the same line of thinking, Rand stipulated that one cannot achieve happiness by wish or whim; there is a heavy emphasis on fulfilling one's own destiny through hard work and a purportedly meritocratic worldview.

Naturally, it's common to see this same approach heralded by many fitness industry individuals. It makes sense—you cannot merely wish for your chest to bulge out proudly underneath the trembling iron of a 100kg back squat, nor should you expect your physique goals—should you have them—to bathe you in unearned glory just by getting out of bed each morning. There is a level of commitment and work required to get from A to B; it doesn't have to be as arduous or "sacrificial" as those unnecessary memes like to proclaim, but consistency is the name of the game when setting out to achieve a goal. For instance, sitting down to write this book requires that I see myself as the creator and nobody else. Nobody else owns the moral impetus to create this book or guarantee its longevity in utility. It is up to me if I want to achieve that satisfaction of sitting down to write and create something and myself alone.

In this sense, the Randian interpretation of happiness has weight in how we navigate not only our fitness goals but life in general. To automatically assume that you are responsible for the vast majority of both positive and negative events in your life can feel a bit narcissistic—you're not omnipotent, after all, and plenty of things remain a mystery to our sense of control, and forever

AYN RAND AND THE OBJECTIVIST FITLOSOPHER

will be—but adopts a position of resilience and adaptivity in the face of adversity.

An Objectivist Fitlosopher, for instance, might be the type of individual who stares at the chaos of the pandemic straight in the eye and decide that they still hold full responsibility for their health and happiness. One may assume this is a somewhat overt position to adopt, considering the ways our brain (or nervous system) responds to stressful events and tries to predict the unpredictable in methods beyond our scope of conscious understanding. A Randian Fitlosopher, naturally, will proclaim that anyone who feels despairing or helpless is simply making excuses—an approach most certainly lacking in empathy and understanding. It appears both sides can learn from one another.

No man is an island.

Rand's philosophy may give us a galvanising kick for getting work done for ourselves, but the assumption that we and we alone are solely responsible for success sets us up for a fall.

Logic dictates that if indeed we are the sole perpetrators for success and achievements, then so it must follow that everything in life that happens to us is our fault. Note that I do not use the term responsibility; the two are markedly different in meaning. It is not our fault, for instance, when we lose a loved one or break a limb; yet to hold this steadfast view so strongly will result in misery and self-loathing.

For one, Objectivist Fitlosophers may accept that any action of success cannot, technically be speaking, be wholly attributed to themselves as beings. They may be able to go to the gym, for instance, but were it not for the business owners, trainers there, and even the people who crafted varying machines and weights, the opportunity to strengthen their bodies would not even exist. Even runs around the neighbourhood constitute some form of contribution from external sources; the trainers on your feet, the gloves, and the leggings were not made by you. Even the money you make that leads to these purchases comes from a long line of factors beyond you in that hour of exercise.

Sure, this seems pedantic—but often, if we are so centred on the self or our own concerns, it can help us to fully expand our perspective on successes and failures. It can really feel like a weight off one's shoulders—Objectivist Fitlosophers are likely to be inexorably hard on themselves if they miss a session or a day's nutrition is less than stellar. When we are more forgiving and gentler on ourselves, we are much more likely to pick ourselves up again after a perceived "blip." In fact, much research in the realms of psychology and therapy treatment today indicates that, on average, people are much more likely to change a habit or behaviour when practicing "self-compassion" regularly. Although there are some qualms as to how one can define such a term and systemise it, it is evident that, on average, there is a negative correlation at the very least between militant attitudes and long-term adherence to habit change. (Note the term *on average*—there will always be exceptions, of course.)

Another way of advocating for flexibility if an individual is struggling with overt Objectivism is counteracting Rand's central flaws with philosophical arguments. If we borrow some of the logic found way back in the Aristotle chapter, we can apply that methodology in uncovering some of the weak spots found in Rand's proposals. In philosophy, we have some things called conditions: logic likes to differentiate between a necessary condition and a sufficient condition.

We have necessary conditions as a means to drive something else to happen or follow through. For example, your house plant will (depending upon how easily killable it is, to your discretion) require water to thrive and survive as a living organism. Yet water is not sufficient to make your house plant grow. Sufficient conditions are sort of like the recipe or blueprint of a statement—they provide all the components required for something to take place. In this instance, a house plant needs soil and a sturdy container in order for it to thrive properly. These are sufficient conditions.

One issue philosophers take with Objectivist arguments is that necessary and sufficient conditions are conflated: Rand assumes that the entrepreneur or solo businessman is a sufficient condition, in that if someone builds a company or starts a new business, then the rest of society falls into place. We need not be philosophers to see that this is evidently not the case. Now there's no doubt in anyone's mind that the aspect of private business fosters economic flourishing. This inevitably leads to societal development and improving the well-being of millions globally. But this still doesn't make it a sufficient condition; rather, we can see that the entrepreneur or what they represent is one of necessity. Still, without economic backing, governmental funding, and even the rules and regulations set into place, which make an individual's goal come into fruition, there can be no budding entrepreneurs to share their contributions in the first place. An Objectivist Fitlosopher might fall into this same trap; exercise goals torment self-development and a better understanding of oneself, that's for certain, but it's not the only thing a human being requires to thrive. Relationships, intellectual development, emotional hygiene, and practical go-to's like shelter or finances all help us lead happy and healthy lives—if not, to exist full stop. Exercise moreover is as much a necessary condition as is the plucky entrepreneur Rand so often lauds.

Rand seems to ignore the fact that happiness and morality, purportedly means of evolutionary survival, are not mutually exclusive terms; since the publishing of her ideas and works, many rotund and robust arguments debunking her claims have been spearheaded in an effort to remind people that being more other-centred has actually demonstrated a significant effect on long-term well-being. Objectivist Fitlosophers, fear not: your sense of emboldened responsibility and hard work is absolutely admirable, but let's not forget the joys life brings when one isn't simply centred on a set goal or stringent routine.

KIERKEGAARD AND THE KIERKEGAARDIAN FITLOSOPHER

Arguably the true granddaddy of the existential school of thought, Kierkegaard offers the contemporary populace both solace and wisdom in the way we understand life's chaotic maelstrom.

Kierkegaard was an interesting fellow during the time of his life (1813–1855). Widely considered to be the first existential philosopher, he noticed a pattern in his philosophical predecessors, in particular, Kant and Hegel: they tended to emphasise the collective, or universality, of human behaviour. Hegel, if you can somehow decipher the utter inanity of his writing, believed that there was a total opposite of what we believed to be knowledge and the ultimate truth. He argues that our thought processes form a component of what it is to be truthful and believes that the goal of pure knowledge can only be attained through awareness of the self, to other "selves" found in humans around us. In short, Hegel (and Kant) loathed the idea of looking to the individual to cultivate a sense of meaning and destiny; he believed it abhorrent as it placed individual good over that of the collective.

Kierkegaard was having none of that, as he believed that there was no real ultimate truth humans had to follow; indeed, he was a philosopher who emphasised the Socratic focus on the individual. He believed that there were ways we could lead authentic lives and hold ourselves to truths beyond that of a collective good, unlike Hegel. As such, we can find much use and relevance in the way we organise our health and fitness, exactly because each and every individual's journeys will manifest differently.

Consider for a moment the context of Kierkegaard's authorial voice. He was born at a time when feudal Denmark was evolving into a society adapted to capitalistic trade, and this also altered the structure of Christendom. Kierkegaard himself was a Christian thinker but disliked the direction the socioeconomic conditions were leading the religious structures of the time. He believed in the importance of carving out an authentic, individual life whilst also considering the grander needs at play across a societal dimension. As a result, he became quite the controversial thinker; his work is spattered with satire, sardonicism, and pseudonyms to lighten the deeper themes discussed within his work.

One of Kierkegaard's bugbears was the church's notion at the time that being an ethically minded individual required little to no effort. Kierkegaard challenged this ideal with his satirical, chameleon-like writings. He asserted that owning a religious faith, specifically that of Christianity, was inexorably challenging to master as a part of one's faith. The ecclesiastical approach implying that leading an ethically sound life was a facile one irked Kierkegaard. He claimed that developing oneself as an individual required struggle and time in order to truly embody a sense of authenticity and personhood.

Kierkegaard created various pseudonyms scattered across his work in order to dilute any kind of bias or assumptions the reader may have when diving into his works. In these pseudonymous works of Kierkegaard, three stages of an individual's lifespan, or rather, three demarcations of how one develops in an existential sense, are outlined: the aesthetic, the ethical, and the religious. It should be noted that Kierkegaard does not suggest a Piaget-like model of developmental stages in a psychological sense. These three stages are, according to Kierkegaard, a naturally intuitive part of each human being. Notably, the "religious" stage revolves mostly around Christian morals and philosophies but need not be confined to the realms of being a pious priest of sorts. Let us discuss, in further detail, what these stages meant to Kierkegaard— and how this applies to an enthused Fitlosopher.

All the World's a Stage

When looking at how Kierkegaard viewed these stages, it's pivotal that we take it one stage at a time. Once more, we must remember that he didn't view these points as chronological or mandatory progressions in the way an individual journeys through their life. Indeed, it's very possible for us to visit and revisit certain stages in a cyclical fashion. There might be times when hedonism feels more important than piety; in a like-minded fashion, periods of indulgence become tiresome, and we resolve ourselves to a more composed way of living.

Though this section is about the Kierkegaardian Fitlosopher, an individual who may assign themselves to this lifestyle-sticking post is likely someone who's been there, done there, got the T-shirt. That's what I enjoy about Kierkegaard's life paths. He doesn't suggest one is more morally "superior" than the other and welcomes fluidity and exploration in the path of an individual's life. An authentic life isn't one that is ethical, stoic, or straightforward; rather, it's messy, comprised of multiple choices, and often involves us reflecting, perhaps even regretting, former actions in order to carve future ones that we take pride in.

The Kierkegaardian Fitlosopher's likely been around the block: fad diets, shoddy attitudes, even downright hating exercise. You name the vice, and they've been there. As such, they'll be sympathetic to Kierkegaard's conception of three life stages. Here, we'll dissect these stages into paths pertaining to fitness and lifestyle change.

The Aesthetic Life Stage: The Fitness Aesthete

The aesthetic stage, according to Kierkegaard, centres itself on hedonism and pleasure; life is made to live, to experience, and nothing is to be taken seriously. Life is, for the aesthete, a thing of immediacy and instant gratification. This is driven by a sort of insatiable drive, whereby each time we fulfill one need, another one crops up in its place. This life stage is about material needs being met, hunting down the satisfaction to our earthly desires.

A Fitness Aesthete might see self-care in the form of Netflix binges, pizza nights, and unleashing the gates of dopamine via online shopping. In effect, it's that quick, pleasurable sensation we do to "treat" ourselves. In the eyes of Kierkegaard, this isn't inherently bad for us, but it's implied from his writings that he considers too much of this, and we become slack and idle in the way we live and think.

Kierkegaard doesn't necessarily exude moral snobbery when setting the scene for an aesthete. Indeed, his existentialist philosophy encourages us to take routes and paths of our own making. Being cajoled into acting like a "moral individual" is merely a form of influence or manipulation by external forces, the exact thing Kierkegaard sought to criticise within the ecclesiastical sector of his time. We are free to carve our own path and make choices based on how our life unravels as a consequence of our actions.

Our actions culminate into a sort of data output. Imagine, for a moment, that our habits, attitudes, worldviews, and daily tasks accumulate to form some kind of graph or chart. We might see, for instance, that 80 percent of our time is spent drinking or watching Netflix. Or that there's a higher daily average of time spent on your phone on the weekend than a Monday evening. These actions inform us of what we truly value despite lip service we may play to impress our confidantes or prospective dates. This data informs us of the ramifications an aesthetic life stage may carry. That we may indeed feel enormous pleasure or gratification at the moment, but by the time that month has run empty, we have little to say for it on a grander scale.

But Kierkegaard believes that the aesthetic stage is an inevitable—note, not compulsory—part of sculpting who we are as individuals. Rather than merely acting as a moral mouthpiece or follower of social norms, we mould our own personal values based on the mistakes and regrets a life of hedonism may bring. A Fitness Aesthete is in the stage of life whereby health and sharpness might be taken for granted. The plucky student, impervious to time's scythe, comes to conjuration. They might mistake the pain or sluggish grinding of consistent work as equivocal to misery. Likewise, slurping a bottle of vodka between rugby bedfellows trumps the euphoria gifted from Manna of the gods.

Priorities are different at this point in an individual's life. It's about embracing life in the moment fully, eschewing routine and recommendations all for a sensory explosion and alternate kind of "presence" that we don't normally correlate mindfulness with. This is the implicit fervor of youthful, free abandon—the objective of each day is not to accumulate meaning but to collect a smorgasbord of beauty, experience, and pleasure. From a rather cynical standpoint, this perspective can be seen as idle-making and pointless. If you see exercise as a cycle of the "sensory reward" experience, no goals or future aspirations are included in the picture; it might look more like a haphazard jogging session after a heavy night out. There's a sense of trying to "feel" the openness of fresh air or getting rid of both physical nausea and emotional embarrassment from a night of hedonism. Food and exercise revolve around pleasure, not purpose.

It is not uncommon for this stage to be a reoccurring stage in a person's life. There's something to be said for the odd bout of escapism. Cognitive psychology is making the link between acts of immersion or numbing and higher self-reported rates of emotional resilience. After all, going full pelt most of the time leaves you in a state of exhausting for double that prescribed period. And each time life throws another wrench in the spanner, we need some kind of emotional backup to provide rejuvenation. Gathering as much experience and exploration in life provides us with strength indirectly. Yet too much in this direction leads to the shirking of responsibility and a sensation of listlessness. One's thought process becomes entirely fixated on satisfying the "now" and how to pleasure oneself, as opposed to taking on the heavy loads of self-sacrifice and cultivating a meaningful living. Pleasure does not equate to enrichment.

Kierkegaard suggests that people quickly tire of this stage. After all, not much can come to fruition when life is orientated solely around instant gratification. Thus, Fitness Aesthetes tend to "grow out" of this period fairly quickly—think of the messy student who suddenly realises that dishes don't magically wash themselves and becomes a responsible housemate overnight. Fitness Aesthetes will go for the quick fix to make themselves good at that moment but not necessarily take on responsibility or goal setting. Thus, Kierkegaardian Fitlosophers appreciate the need for this life period in order for them to understand and appreciate structure and purpose. This is where the ethical life stage comes in.

The Ethical Life Stage: The Fitness Ethicist

The Fitness Ethicist embodies the total opposite of the aesthetic life stage. Unlike the aforementioned, life is nothing but serious choices for the Fitness Ethicist. According to Kierkegaard, the ethical stage suggests that life is truly what you make of it. All to say: your choices, your actions, mould the path your life paves out. It is not enough to merely live—or experience pleasure, as aestheticism may argue—but to make honest choices that give life to your existence; to how you view your sense of self, in other words.

A Fitness Ethicist might be a stickler for strict goals and specific routines, for instance, interloping them with personal values and how they see themselves. Fitness is an honour and responsibility for the ethicist: to not move your body or eat in a way that encourages sluggishness or reticence would be to semi-betray your own sense of being. It sounds fairly melodramatic, and Kierkegaard actually notes this as a critique against the (overall wholesome) image of the ethicist. Just doing something because it "seems" like the proper, right thing to do is not necessarily carving out an individual stake for oneself. It's following social mores and values besieged by others before them.

But overall, Kierkegaard keeps his lips sealed when it comes to punitive judgment. All of mankind, after all, may visit these stages at least once in their lives. And so, a Fitness Ethicist might have grown weary of a life filled with hedonism and ill-built structure. It may creep up on the same in the same transcendent, ecclesiastical glory that the slap of a self-help book beams across one's face in the stinging dawn of a recent breakup. A person might wake up and suddenly desire transformation, goals, or achievement. The aesthetic life stage offers enjoyment and sensory fulfillment, sure, but cannot attend to one's needs in the same capacity as an ethical life approach.

The ethical life stage can coincide with or proceed directly beyond that of the aesthetic. What is notable is that it takes precedence over the choice of the instantaneous. When faced with a decision based around hedonistic, gratifying desire and societal obedience, the latter will prevail. It's a bit like when a student gets invited to the hottest party of the year or to stay in the library before a serious exam the following day; the ethicist will acknowledge an existence of pleasurable desire but conclude that the best course of action is to subordinate these yearnings. The aesthetic life has no coherent, existing framework for what is deemed to be "good." One cannot live for others if the pursuit of a "good life" is solely orientated around what sways away boredom and the pangs of banality. The ethical life stage, on the other hand, is proposed by Kierkegaard as a means to construct a set of norms and attitudes which promotes social cohesion and overarching concern of welfare for others. In other words, the Fitness Ethicist does things not for some sweet rush of pleasure, but because the choices and actions they take invoke sets of principles to live a life beyond their own sense of self.

A Fitness Ethicist will be forced to take these choices when faced with the option of indulging in frivolous, present-day shenanigans versus a greater, collective "good." This "good," according to

Kierkegaard, is one molded by societal norms and expectations, based around putting others before the self. In this instance, nourishing oneself appropriately and getting exercise might not be the easiest thing in the world. Yet it sets the standard for the way we view others by proxy of how we treat ourselves. If we treat our own bodies and minds as means rather than ends, we cannot afford to respect ourselves. And if we are unable to respect ourselves, it stands to reason that showing up for others to support them becomes a sluggishly proportioned task.

The Religious Life Stage: The Fitness...Christian?

As can be deduced by this piece, Kierkegaard wasn't the biggest fan of Hegelian philosophy. In fact, whilst Hegel was one to assume that ethics were the highest order of living our lives, Kierkegaard chose the 4D-chess route and tackled this proposal with his own rebuttal. In one of his masterpieces, *Fear and Trembling*, Kierkegaard argues on behalf of a third category—a category that transcended the materialist concepts, anchored by human ethics, and was a required part of exploring who we are in the existentialist sense of the term. This category is known as the religious life stage.

For Kierkegaard, the religious life stage is the highest form of living. In other words, it's the stage in which individuals are able to live on their own terms as opposed to abiding by the parroting of others' advice. In *Fear and Trembling*, Kierkegaard uses the biblical story of Abraham being asked by God to sacrifice his son, Isaac, to highlight this point. (Yes, it seems gross and a little out there. But keep following.) By contemporary standards, it's pretty clear that

Abraham needed a parenting book or two before sticking to his decision. I might not be a mother, but I'm fairly sure that according to some as-of-yet-proven sky deity's wish to murder your son falls under the umbrella of "parenting no-nos." In terms of biblical symbolism and literary prowess, however, his story is a powerful one. Abraham's willingness to adhere to God's word and kill his son (to clarify, there was a happy ending: no biblical story figures were harmed in the making of this moral lesson) was a decision so drastic that it could only be considered a "leap of faith."

From any perspective but that of faithful living, Abraham's decision is clearly bewildering. Plus, it also sets the bar pretty low by most parenting standards today. Yet this disbarring of our own ethical preconceptions and societal attitudes has a place in Kierkegaard's interpretation. It is known as the "teleological suspension of the ethical," as it is with faith that Abraham exerts his willingness to make his own decisions, notwithstanding the extrinsic judgments toward his actions. Naturally, this is a drastic example for Kierkegaard to demarcate (surely by now you'd have figured he's got a flair for the dramatic?) but the point stands quite strongly.

The teleological suspension of the ethical is a bit of a mouthful and difficult to deconstruct. But there's a way we can review it without allowing our brains to implode.

Say, for instance, you're walking down the street, and your stomach starts mewling at you in hunger and Sunday afternoon despair. If you are hungry, it's only sensible that you scroll through foodporn across Deliveroo for your next meal, with the goal of no longer being hungry. This is the definition of a teleological decision: you acted, by eating or ordering, so as to achieve the end of no longer experiencing tummy grumbles.

In *Fear and Trembling*, Abraham performs a *teleological suspension of the ethical* the moment he decides to sacrifice Isaac. Abraham knows that killing Isaac is unethical the same way he knows the sky is blue. However, Abraham decides to suspend the ethical. In other words, he puts his ethical concerns about killing his son on the back burner; his faith that righteousness and a higher truth will be achieved is the thing that trumps these woes. Abraham's faith that God would never allow an unethical means allows him to undertake what appears to be an unethical decision. Abraham puts religious concerns over ethical concerns, thus taking a leap of faith and living life on terms beyond earthly anxieties.

It should be of note that Kierkegaard specifies the religious doctrine of Christianity—hence the particular label.

Kierkegaard's attack on the Danish church was based on his concern the religious figures of the time chose to prescribe "goodness" and morality onto the people rather than having them figure out for themselves what constitutes leading an ethical life.

Kierkegaard's religious stage acknowledges the futility in creating this perfect, godly-like self attempted through the ethical life stage. Through taking a leap in faith, much like Abraham, you accept and embrace your imperfect nature as a human being and live your life authentically. There's no staunch responsibility nor senseless pleasure. There's a sense of bestowing to yourself an inner peace of who you are as a human being, a trust that something greater beyond your current means will lead to a transcendent end.

That's not to say the religious stage is apathetic towards ethical living. Kierkegaard was a Christian, so it makes sense that his writing might sway toward the more meaningful paths of living. Specifically, he begs the question: what makes something meaningful for an individual? What makes a person choose a particular path, to get up each day and work, day by day, toward something a little bit greater than themselves?

Okay, you've pelted me with philosophy. What gives now? Why Kierkegaard?

I must confess: I have a soft spot for Kierkegaard as a thinker. Much of his points merit our attention as cosmopolitan inhabitants, our thoughts are regularly strewn across the floor in an array of existential confetti. There will always be periods of our lives when we feel angst-ridden or paralysed by the ache of regret, the "what ifs" that hack into our taut vault of consciousness as we stare up at the ceiling before bedtime.

This is why knowing who we are and what we stand for is so damn important, particularly when we are attempting to create or mold a new lifestyle. Following someone else's values on what they conceive to be worth pursuing is a recipe for disaster and personal misery. If you're someone who loves the thrill of chasing a new lifting PB and you're adhering to the fluid openness of a regular yoga practice, your skin will be crawling with the itch of impatience and frustration. In a similar vein, a new mum just wanting to find five minutes' worth of routine in her maelstrom of a day would find no joy in exercise if they were given a six-week bodybuilding programme.

The Kierkegaardian Fitlosopher respects this. They understand the need for human individuality and uncovering one's own personal values and boundaries. Core values help us aim to achieve a greater transcendence than dolloping peanut butter into our oats every Monday. Our own bespoke values help us understand what we need out of our lives better.

Now, Kierkegaard never suggested there was an "ultimate truth," nor did he imply one was better than the other. He simply outlined these three stages as choices. We may dally in each stage at certain times of our lives, and each path may serve us well for that time. And that's perfectly okay. What's important is that we make a choice—it's us and us alone who decide how to live. We must discover for ourselves which path truly connects to our values for a fulfilling, meaningful life.

Kierkegaardian Fitlosophers may boast this sense of openness, a reverence or respect for the nuance required to respect our human condition.

How open is too open?

The notion of being "too open" is an issue that has plagued philosophers and psychologists alike for centuries. Attempts at exploring and explaining human behaviour have been made from any and all corners of the academic battlefield. Some argue that personality emerges as a purely biological phenomenon, almost acting as a kind of primal driver into the way we interpret information around us. Ironically enough, this deterministic worldview—despite purporting itself to follow an evidence, science-based blueprint— follows the cocaine-laced footsteps of Sigmund Freud, perhaps unknowingly. Psychoanalysts such as Sigmund Freud and later Carl Jung purported that human beings were driven toward a set of behaviours that were essentially ensconced within our own fears, desires, and needs. In other words, behaviour for these thinkers was a **nomothetic** phenomenon.

Nomothetic is a word that stems from the Greek origin "nomos," otherwise translated generically as "law." In psychology, the term is used to define a type of study that seeks to cultivate objective knowledge or data, and by doing so, formulate laws that apply to everyone. The field of cognitive psychology is a form of nomothetic study, for instance, because it attempts to create frameworks in the way we understand how humans learn and memorise things.

Kierkegaardian Fitlosophers are not one for definitives nor extremes. The individual, for them, predates any type of collectivist wisdom. So, a nomothetic approach wouldn't behoove their values; for them, the individual is prioritised. This has its obvious advantages. One is at a far lower risk of falling prey to generalised plans, which harbour little consideration toward personal preference. Therein lies the rub: a lack of objectivity can instigate failure to commit to a given decision or principle.

When an individual has a concrete goal, it is important to maintain a degree of flexibility in the method of attaining it. Dietary approaches are a practical example of this. If we take the basic adage of calories in, calories out, we understand that any given human physiology cannot defy the basic tenets of physics. That is to say: in order to lose or gain weight, we have to consume more or fewer calories, respectively. The goal is cemented, but the methodologies of getting there can vary.

This might be the core values of the Kierkegaardian Fitlosopher surmised into one neat package.

If we imagine his stages to be arranged in a format that's less verbose, we'd arrive at the sensible conclusion of a Venn diagram. Both Ethical and Aesthetic sandwich the Religious stage. In effect, the Religious stage takes the individual from the Aesthetic and the collective from the Ethical to create a hybrid. Kierkegaard Fitlosophers snug themselves nicely into this hybrid; there's a respect, an acknowledging toward the empirical importance of calorie intake. Yet better still these individuals know there's more than one way to skin a cat. Both a higher-carb, lower-fat diet and a lower-carb, higher-fat diet extoll virtues in and of themselves: research points to higher energy levels amongst varying individuals for both. Lower carb diets, for instance, have been anecdotally associated with improved focus, whilst carb-loading during the evening is linked to improved sleep. These perks, of course, run alongside the capacity to tweak any given caloric intake dependent on a goal. Regardless of whether you choose the path of a ritualistic caveman or litter your kitchen with cornflakes, the message is clear: fitness and nutrition outcomes are not determined by one sole path.

Now, the Kierkegaardian Fitlosopher understands this nuance perfectly well, to a fault: running the gauntlet of a "grey area" or "nuance" may lead to a flip-flop of focus. An individual's actions and habits must line up somewhat to any given desired goal. Research indicates that habit change is one of accumulative, subtle change; in other words, small yet consistent actions over time trump grandiose tweaks. Much of our present-day behaviour may stem from things that we have "learnt," be it from the people around us or societal constructs that wedge us in. Why do we pursue certain situations or dynamics, for instance, if they only serve to codify low levels of self-esteem or worth? Why do we unconsciously undertake specific habits? What do these actions signify to us about the way we view ourselves? The individual, in some cases, does indeed trump age-old wisdom. Yet if a person is chopping and changing their habits more than a pinball chops and changes its trajectory, this can lead to them stagnating or being stuck at square one.

Tempting as it is to abscond traditional wisdom over the individual, there are some unavoidable, grounded truths that another individual, like a Marxist Fitlosopher, might choose to favour. Data, numerical findings, and the overall scientific method are necessary tenets in understanding human physiology. So, we cannot always die on the hill on nuance if we are to exact and improve performance. This is one hurdle the Kierkegaardian Fitlosopher must overcome: to be decisive in their desires based upon logical rationale, rather than hovering over numerous options.

Not that there's anything inherently "wrong" about having a bespoke approach toward human behaviour. The idiographic model can prove to be as useful a tool as any in understanding ourselves and why we behave the way we do. As those psychotherapists of old understand, processing one's own human experience is an integral part of becoming a wholly adaptive human being. Based on their own experiences, sociocultural surroundings, and neurobiology, an individual sitting opposite from you on the train to work may have an entirely different blueprint of what constitutes success, well-being, or health; it would do you no good to follow their footsteps. This lies at the heart of a Kierkegaardian Fitlosopher's lifestyle, and when employed properly, serves people well.

Still, a sample size of one is an unacceptable reference point when underpinning scientific concepts. Quantitive, empirical hypotheses about the human brain and body are informative; without concrete examples as to how the nervous system responds to stimuli, for instance, I as a coach cannot give clients a suitable framework to improve their well-being. It can feel intuitive, albeit solipsistic, to rely solely on what "feels" right. Ironically, despite Kierkegaard's philosophy opposing postmodernism's tenets, there appears to be a "snake eating its own" phenomenon occurring between the two ideologies. Much like the Postmodernist Fitlosopher, these individuals might prioritise lived experience above empirical data. This is all well and good for fostering bespoke plans, but when it comes at the cost of tenable achievements, the Kierkegaardian might hit a wall. If they plan on competing in their first powerlifting meet but believe their programming should consist primarily of yoga and breathwork on the basis of enjoyment, therein lies conflict. Inevitably, satisfaction and meaning wane in the long run. Even when examining the original philosophy, some argue that Kierkegaard's conception of the religious life stage comes at a price: boredom and angst. It is finding the reprieve from this anxiety that underpins much of Kierkegaard's concepts. Yet if a person engages in habits that have no consolidating root in material results, then no matter how validating it is for their personal preferences, this sense of listlessness cannot be remedied.

The frivolities of considering one's existential purpose in daily living is a luxury Kierkegaard and others could afford. When we're nipping out to get more milk or scouring out a tube seat on a Monday morning, such opportunities for contemplation are ill-afforded. Considering too much of "why" someone does something just leads to rumination, with little action entailed. Sometimes, then, it makes sense for the Kierkegaardian Fitlosopher to step back and trust the process set forth by falsifiable—or reputable—scientific methods. Examining the methods of deduction showcased by Marxist, or even Randian, Fitlosophers might prove prudent for the average Angsty Joe who tends to have their head in the clouds.

ALBERT CAMUS AND THE ABSURDIST FITLOSOPHER

It's a truth universally acknowledged (unfortunately) that philosophy on the whole is not exactly considered the sexiest field of study to immerse oneself.

Cue Albert Camus, hater of monogamy and lover of large boulders, being pushed up hills.

Camus is often categorised as an existentialist. And perhaps if we were layman about it, you might be right. But Camus sought to expand the school of existentialism, as he was virulently opposed to most structural or systemic schools of philosophy. (Natch, he was a total rebel without a cause.) He proposed almost a subset of existentialism, known as absurdism.

Camus begins with the Aristotelian question that most humans have pondered at least once upon a drunken evening. What is the meaning of our existence? In a similar vein to existentialists, Camus argues that no such thing exists. Camus acknowledges that humans are inclined to quest and yearn for such an answer, yet the irresolvable truth is that the universe remains silent and apathetic toward our angst. We must, therefore, learn to accept or process this lack of meaning in our lives. Camus dubbed the paradox between searching for a sense of meaning in a meaning-less universe and the impossibility of fulfilling said emptiness the absurd. Absurdism thus explores the gap between our own desire to cultivate meaning in a meaningless universe and how we try to bridge it by finding purpose in, say, making a cup of coffee.

One of Camus' best-known philosophical works is *The Myth of Sisyphus*, in which he delves into this idea further by focusing on the Greek myth itself. Sisyphus was an unfortunate (or fortunate, Camus may argue) man who was punished by the gods and sent for all eternity to push a boulder up a mountain, only for it to roll all the way back down again, ready for Sisyphus to commence the climb again.

Sounds sucky, I know. But Camus contended that this perpetuity of mediocre activity is the secret sauce to happiness. As long as Sisyphus accepts—perhaps, fully embraces—the absurd struggle and lifelong, mundane task set before him, he can find sincere happiness and meaning in the meaninglessness. As the famed aphorism goes: *"One must imagine Sisyphus happy."*

An Absurdist Fitlosopher might be a funny one, but they certainly exist out there. The notion of having to start to attend the gym, then not actually having a finish line or set endpoint, can feel terrifying and imitate much self-doubt or confusion about one's goals. An Absurdist Fitlosopher might be the existential one of the bunch to note that, no, commencing a relationship with exercise or improved nutrition is not a one-stop-shop. It's likely we'll all have to go to the gym for the rest of our human lives, lest we become sloth-like, depressed, or lose that confident gleam a brand-new pair of well-fitting jeans may bring.

An individual hyper-focused on meaning and goals, for instance, will feel the lull of frustration each time a hurdle is met or a goal is ticked off. You may have seen these examples in people you know. You may even recognise a few in your own life.

1. "My New Year's resolution is to lose all my Christmas weight. Then, I can relax a bit more."
2. "Once I've gotten a bit fitter, I'll feel more confident in myself."
3. "I have a couple of dress sizes to lose. Then I'll be free, and I can stop killing myself at the gym!"

The Absurdist Fitlosopher and embracing the absurdity of wearing lycra three to five times a week.

Humans are confronted with the notion of banality every day of their waking lives.

Think about it. When somebody asks you, "How was your day?" the only honest and accurate evaluation would be, on average, "My day was fine." Very rarely, unless tragic or miraculous or downright strange outliers occur, do our days differ in any particular way. Our work routines are set, often meeting the same people and engaging in similar activities from the day before.

(Sorry. I'm essentially outlining the depressing reality that is life. I really am a philosopher now, I guess.)

In short: very little do our days differentiate or demarcate anything remarkable on a regular basis. We are confined by the framework we have created, which can either be asphyxiating or empowering.

It might feel this way, attending to your gym sessions and programming week in, week out, with little to no variation save the numbers on the plates or the adjustments prescribed every few weeks. An Absurdist Fitlosopher will face this banality in the eye and accept it for what it is. They will be more likely to find the exciting or positive or meaningful in the face of the meaningless; each session offers itself up as a foundation for something greater, in what appears to be a maelstrom of routine and vapidity.

A philosopher like Nietzsche was similar in Camus' vein of thinking but differed in his conclusions. Nietzsche proposed that the great artifices of everyday living—art, poetry, literature, and music—were things that gave the apathy of life some kind of meaning, despite being an illusory force. By this metric, we could essentially become the artists—or, to paraphrase Nietzsche, the poets—of our lives.

Camus is, frankly, more brutally honest (if you follow his line of thinking that there is no objective meaning or morality constructed in our world) in the sense that he disagrees with dressing up our banal routine with sugary lies. For Camus, the "absurd hero" takes no refuge in the illusions procured by the arts, religion, or literature—yet neither does he just pack it all in with glib despair. Sisyphus is, according to Camus, the archetypal absurd hero in that he openly embraces the absurdity of his situation. He fully recognises the futility and uselessness of rolling his boulder up the mountain, only to repeat the task for all eternity. Yet in his actions, he remains present, willing, and able.

Weirdly, it's precisely this honest acceptance of the grim truth in front of us which forms the solution to what Camus hypothesises as the source of human existential angst. We are able to look at this futility dead in the eye whilst refusing to let the grim truth destroy our lives. It's arguably more poetic than using actual poetry to buttress our ways of living.

It might not be the most comforting thought in the world, is it? How exactly does confronting the absurdity of Sisyphus' absurd situation give him a reason to keep going?

But maybe it's not supposed to be comforting.

Maybe it's all there is.

An Absurdist Fitlosopher acknowledges this. They recognise that despite the apparent futility and inane routine of attending their gym sessions until death do they part, there is a grit and character-building element in denying one's own rejection of reality; if we were to continually fight and resist against the fact we require a healthy standard of living to accommodate our own self-respect and physiological well-being, then we'd probably live a very miserable life indeed. Which is somewhat of a bitter cherry on the top of a life devoid of meaning, right?

Is there meaning in the madness of it all? Or are Absurdist Fitlosophers bang on?

There is an erstwhile resilience in the attitude of the Absurdist Fitlosopher: no matter the task, no matter how arduous, they'll be the ones to plod along, knowing that in doing so and embracing their task, they are fulfilling a destiny greater than the empty path the universe sets before them.

Oddly, their deference to an apathetic universe means they'll likely be the ones to get in daily habits. They'll likely be the ones to see food as something that fuels their activities and gets to a greater goal. The goal itself may not be representative, necessarily, of something bigger than themselves, but as they are not shying away from this potential lack of thing-ness, they end up cultivating a microcosmic universe of their own, full of meaning.

Picture an ice cream shop. You walk in, your eyes hit by a smorgasbord and colours you never thought to exist; flavours that appeared concocted by the whims of a mad scientist. You say to your friend that there are no other ice cream shops down the street; happily, this small business seems to have procured itself a real niche. There's no other way of choosing any other flavours, beyond those that are set before you. You can, however, despite these restrictions, choose any flavour you like in said cosy gelateria; you just can't go beyond the framework of the ice cream shop and pick anything else.
This analogy has been used in many **free-will** arguments, especially by thinkers such as Daniel Dennett in his approach to the philosophy of mind. Essentially, he argues that despite us having no true volition or control beyond the remit of our evolved brains and that we must depend on how our minds develop in instilling morality within us, we can indeed choose our actions in a set framework.
I enjoy this analogy, too, when trying to explain the idea of creating meaning when none appears to exist. We may not be able to walk out of the ice cream shop (our own universe, or at least, a conception of what is there) of our own will and find external meaning, but we can pick the flavours in the closed quarters of an ice cream shop (the world that appears to us as it is) in order to carve out a sort of artificial purpose.

It's worth noting, of course, that living a life devoid of perceived meaning appears pretty groovy at first: there's no objective sticking post you must adhere to. Everything, technically speaking, becomes relative. If nothing in our experience of the world matters, fitness included, then all bets are off: we could technically do anything, and according to Camus, cultivate a meaning of our own and assign it to an activity.

Which, y'know, includes stuff like Netflix binging. Late nights playing PS4. Maybe some cocaine.

Okay, fine, the cocaine example seems a little extreme, but the point remains: if nothing matters in our universe, and technically speaking, we can cultivate any kind of purpose in all sorts of activities. At face value, this is pretty great: we've no risk of boredom or complaining about quotidian actions, like attending the gym or resisting the urge to stuff our faces with pizza every meal of the day.

The issue is this: if we can be so quick to assign our own acceptance of discipline and routine in their mundanity, we can do the same with the exact opposite set of values. Suddenly, spending all day in bed doing nothing but watching *Tiger King* and eating Krispy Kreme has inherent meaning. (And, for the record, I'm not saying a duvet-doughnut day is a bad thing—quite the opposite. The poison is in the dosage.) Suddenly, as the universe is apathetic and has no purpose, we become less selective in what we view to be worth pursuing. The act of assigning meaning to something is facile and quick. Because if nothing is objectively "meaningful," why not go the whole hog and swap mundane discipline for hedonistic pleasure?

An Absurdist Fitlosopher, as a result, has to take Camus' worldview with a pinch of salt. If they think it's simply a case of "getting on with it" and taking it day by day—because really, what else is there—they must try and use empirical, measurable factor analyses to not let their boulder run down the hill, beyond control, causing chaos in the form of nightly pub visits.

This could be checking daily steps, weekly measurements, or weigh-ins, and just checking in on their gym progress, in general, to ensure they're getting from A to B, despite views on its inanity.

Another thing worth noting is that thinkers have often associated meaning and purpose with pain. An Absurdist Fitlosopher could easily look at life's distresses straight in the eye and deny them outright, labelling them as purposeless and innocuous. If we took this meaning quite literally, could we really outright say that we can derive little to no meaning in our fitness strives? Generally speaking, when we start lifting or running, the exercise feels pretty horrible, and we view ourselves as rather weak. As time wears on, we notice the ebb and dilution of crusty muscle soreness or desperate gasps for air; we are able to compare the pain we experience now to what we felt then. A disparity might, in some cases, indicate a heightened level of fitness and thus greater steps accrued to one's goal in the first place—a pretty meaningful feat.

It would, therefore, be prudent for the average Absurdist Fitlosopher to acknowledge that Camus' view has limitations, in that we as humans naturally intuit some form of meaning in our lives—no matter how artificial, false, or illusory it may seem to be. Sometimes, it's best to throw caution to the wind—and rock to the bottom of the hill—and embrace the non-empirical sentimentality life has to offer, savour its aesthetic freedom, and realise that it's okay to construct purpose that isn't borne from apathy or non-belief.

STOICISM AND
THE STOIC FITLOSOPHER

For those of you who might be living under a rock or Plato's Cave, Stoicism is arguably the most pronounced and promoted school of philosophy amidst the meme-ing thresholds of social media.

From Ryan Holiday to Lewis Howes, there hasn't been a modern-day popular thinker who hasn't touched upon the words uttered by Seneca, Aurelius, or Epictetus, albeit in ways that might make the aforementioned philosophers frown a little. (That's not to say my attempts will be any better, but it's worth noting that the original texts and tenets from the lofty Stoic giants contain much more pith and vigour than any of those self-help books and my own series could ever muster.)

And there's a good reason for it. Stoicism is often attributed to a deeper, ingrained, almost intuitive wisdom deep within us that guides us to lead better lives and abstain from emotionally charged decisions. They contributed to formal structures of logic and theories of causality, which ended brilliantly with how they viewed self-responsibility and the events surrounding our actions.

Contrary to popular belief, Stoicism is not about repressing emotions or disregarding them; rather, actively choosing to behave in a certain way despite the rampant urge to key your ex's car or scream in the ear of a nefarious slow walker. Whilst you'll likely hear the names above in any tome referencing Stoicism, it's important to fully outline its origins. Socrates had a massive influence on Zeno of Citium's thought process, and eventually, his ideas began the spark of debate that turned into an academic forest fire across Athens and then the entirety of Rome.

And it became not only a practical, scholarly way of living but self-referential in its premise, too. Aurelius allegedly wrote his works to remind himself of the tenets promoted by stoicism, mentally equipping himself with the basic ideals that his fellow thinkers would advise him. This is often the reason readers purport his work to be aphoristic or sloganeering, "Erase impressions" and "Do nothing at random." Aurelius wrote his meditations for his own moral improvement. Reminders that happiness is a virtue to be practiced and is wholly in an individual's control can be easily applied to life's strife and general goal-setting.

There's a great deal of popular Stoic philosophers currently being read voraciously, so this section will do its best to summarise and relate their ideas to the average Fitlosopher's way of thinking. There's only so many black-and-white Instagram quotes I can wade through and analyse, after all.

What's so great about these guys, anyway?

Stoicism has made waves in terms of both historical and contemporary forms of impact. We see it today, for example, in schools of psychotherapy such as Cognitive Behavioural Therapy. It acts as a form of virtue ethics in that thinkers espoused the need to practice traits and mannerisms in order to lead a happy life. For instance, health is not naturally granted to you; one would need to exert effort and decision-making in what they eat and how they train. Stoicism is considered to be a **Hellenistic eudaemonic philosophy**—in very simple terms, the Stoics took heavy influence from Socrates, Aristotle, and early Platonic dialogues. They sought to examine the values and meaning derived from life's activities as a way of accepting the frustrations we face as a whole. It comes as no surprise, therefore, that there's a massive overlap between these schools of thinking.

The idea of Stoicism is that we expand upon our psychological toolkit, developing inner calm, clear judgment, and freedom from suffering. Our feelings and emotions are all valid and healthy, but Stoicism aims to temper our reactions to them in an effort to lead a better quality of life. Thus, Stoicism becomes a way of life: it engages with self-dialogue, contemplation of our mortality, and advocation of the present moment.

As an approach to fitness, Stoicism isn't half bad; I'd even err on the side of making it a prerequisite to season a bit of this mind-set into one's own approach, regardless of whichever Fitlosophy branch you find yourself slotting into. The reason being, Stoicism as a school of thought emphasises the practical need to deal with life's blows in a way that fosters resilience and acceptance; Epictetus, for instance, a well-known proponent of the philosophy, was once himself a slave, so likely knows better than anyone the benefits of acceptance and embracing the painful.

So does that mean Stoic Fitlosophers just don't care? Like at all?

One of the more common misconceptions floating about the generic analyses of Stoicism is that the thinkers who advocated for it just didn't "care" or were in favour of repressing emotions rather than accepting or honouring them. Indeed, it certainly doesn't help that our contemporary vernacular has tweaked the term Stoicism to befit our linguistical needs; the word is now associated with stiff upper lips and emotionally stunted Joe Rogan guests. The philosophy, however, says nothing about denial or stuffing away the pains of life; rather, its focus is on reframing and reexamining tough situations in order to walk away with dignity and strength intact.

That we can endure arduous situations is not mutually exclusive to feeling sucky about what's going on, either.

Stoic Fitlosophers will, in all likelihood, have a natural intuition that training and movement transcend vanity, translating instead to discipline and mindset outside of the gym.

A Stoic Fitlosopher may have a better understanding that we are in control of ourselves. External woes, rather than paralysing us and preventing growth, enables us with resilience and empowerment. When you are aware that the world itself cannot be changed, but you can, odds are you're going to work a bit harder to find better at navigating situations like social or work drinks and busy travel schedules.

Stoic Fitlosophers, as a result, share this common wisdom that some things in our life just refuse to bend to our will. We can hope that loved ones don't get sick as much as we want; it doesn't mean we guarantee their safety. We can be kind and good to others all day long, without any guarantee that this principle of charity will be returned. As Epictetus notes, "We are responsible for some things, while there are others for which we cannot be held responsible."

From the perspective of neuroscience, Stoicism holds some truths that remain deeply ingrained in the psyche of growth mindset and emotional resilience. The brain is essentially a "prediction organ," as aptly stated by Professor Andrew Huberman, a neurobiologist based at Stanford University, and will constantly seek out ways to determine the duration of a stressful circumstance, the path required in order to reach a solution, and ultimately to decipher an outcome and uncover what exactly will occur at the end of this process.

These three paths tackled all at once, transmogrify into sullen Cerberus heads, guarding the path toward unknown ventures and future success. It's wise to choose one path, or one way of "predicting," as it were, rather than try to tackle all three at once. In a sense, then, when Stoics mention how only some things are in our control, on a neurophysiological level, this might be what they'd be referring to our brilliant yet bewildering brains only able to juggle a certain number of tasks at a time, with the rest becoming static, heavy noise in the background. It's wise to pick your battles when it comes to habit change and start small, or you risk creating more unnecessary cognitive load to your worldly experience than before you started.

All to say, our brains dislike large upheavals in routine. It indicates a threat or veering away from what is known to be stable and certain. It's why habit change is best approached with baby steps and a cautious eye, just carefully observing your physiological responses to introducing a new change into your life.

Are you feeling resistant? Stressed? Tense? Good, this is the gateway to dopaminergic pathways doing the work and eventually, finally giving you that "good feeling" we associate with reward and meaning. That initial resistance going into a new task is not only normal but inevitable if we are to garner any neurochemical benefit from the action: it is, in essence, the brain assessing its new stimulus and environmental change and adjusting to it.

Modern-day neuroscience, by chance, finds kinship with the intuitive wisdom espoused by thinkers of the Stoic school of philosophy. Thinkers like Aurelius and Epictetus, two individuals who themselves found worldly experience in enduring great duress (though, I think the latter "won out" this category by proxy of his unwilling serfdom), believed in experiencing that mental fog, that emotional sluggishness we experience by monotony and pain. Whilst we may not be emperors taking risky decisions or being forced into slavery, we commonly experience or note the "hardness" of daily routine.

The "hardness" of going to the gym and eating vegetables when you just want to stay in bed. The "hardness" of finishing a project when the mental softness of watching a Netflix series feels so, so good. The "hardness" of undertaking habit changes when current living feels soporific or comfortable.

Stoic Fitlosophers recognise that difficulty and strife are parts of our lives and unavoidable. But we can choose our hard. We might think that choosing pleasure and the hedonic sensation of sugar, fat, and booze-laced nights out (or in, as 2020 has dictated, nights in with a side of self-hatred) feels better than a painful, boring, arduous weight session; or that "adult food" cannot trump the sensory joys begotten by grease or creaminess or salted crunching, but that is a short-lived, superficial jolt of gratification as opposed to the unbeatable feeling of victory over the self.

It is far harder, overall, to live a life without any pursuit of the meaningful or goals greater than our daily living. It is far harder to know that you may not be adept at keeping your own word to yourself. Stoics believed that these levels of difficulty were far more corrosive than slogging through an hour or adhering to a sensible diet.

Are Stoic Fitlosophers the "Ideal"?

I would err on the side of caution when suggesting any one approach is the Adonis of mental or emotional sharpening—we are, after all, wondrously, gloriously varied individuals who have had different upbringings, have goopy grey matter consisting of different genetic makeups, and experience a whole host of various experiences that cannot exactly match another's.

The world is an immensely complex, rich, and often terrifying place; far too, complexity is preferred to us, for instance, and an endless number of phenomena are put out on display for us to perceive, understand and assimilate. One of the biggest problems humans face is this perception and assimilation of the information presented in front of us. In some sense, we attempt to "simplify" this sensory overwhelm (and try to get out of bed without having an existential breakdown) by using apt filters or schemas that enable us to interact with the environment—and people—around us.

Because the world is so full and complex, one of the biggest issues we have to attempt to solve as human beings is how we see things around us and act in a way that is both significant and meaningful. Stoicism, at least the way I see it, is an exceptionally efficient philosophy in a way that embodies this ideal of assimilation and action; it's a wholly practical philosophy. It offers people a set of practical and accessible emotional toolkits for us to make our navigation around this world maximally useful.

This mysterious conglomerate of worldly complexity and the richness, the infuriating and nauseating richness of the human condition, it goes without saying that a moderated, stoic approach may not marry well with everyone. And this is perfectly okay. There also tends to be a somewhat tenuous link (I say "tenuous" as an N=1 observer here) between the Stoic school of thought and its conflation with repression of emotion. If you find you are an individual who harbours avoidant tendencies or who struggles with emotional vulnerability, tread cautiously in the way you integrate Stoicism into your daily routine; it may be that a philosophy based more upon spontaneity or embracing one's emotions in the face of life's inanity, such as absurdism or existentialism, might be more prudent for your own development.

In terms of philosophical rebuttal, some thinkers argue that Stoicism is a hyper-physicalist approach to navigating the world. In other words, they miss the forest for the trees in favour of hardened logic. The latter can indeed be enormously helpful when understanding or diluting intense emotions but taken too far, it wrongly supposes the purpose or meaning behind our feelings. Integrity, love, and desire are metaphysical concepts that cannot be accounted for by mere physicalist approaches. Further to this, a Stoic Fitlosopher might become rather rigid in their ordering of the world, and as such, their relationship with the environment around them may manifest in such a way that socialising and exploratory, open phases with food and exercises become shunned in favour of routine and a perceived "wisdom." It becomes akin to the Kantian line of thinking in that if they set a value they perceive to be an integral part of how they manifest themselves and their goals in the world, that value becomes practically unbreakable, a part of themselves. It might be prudent for the Stoic Fitlosopher at times to appreciate the hedonism and carefree acts that eschew the composed, moderate life many of their go-to thinkers might advocate for. Moments, glimpses of the hedonic become reminders for the Stoic Fitlosopher as to exactly *why* they prefer the sturdy doldrums of routine, programmed training schedules, and plates adorned with vegetation aplenty; sure, a binge-watch of *Schitt's Creek* coupled with a

Domino's pizza (or two) might feel good at that moment but that moment only. The indulgence becomes an occasional escapist form of adventure in its own right, rather than a continual path to chaos and listlessness some nihilistic attitudes may convey.

It is only by experiencing this chaos that the Stoic Fitlosopher will come to truly appreciate why they abide by the values and philosophies they do, rather than be tempted to make said mozzarella orgy a weekly regular. Someone who is profoundly embedded in the Stoic mentality may benefit from being a wee bit selfish or hedonistic: looking toward some form of extrinsic motivation, as studies have shown, can fuel us with the fire we need to kick it up a notch.

It might help bolster praise or respect from others, earn them prestige in a sport they practice or even help them attain a goal weight. None of these aims are particularly Stoic but certainly have their place in the whirligig of the human psyche.

Are you perhaps a bit too Stoic in this modern-day hullaballoo, or do you think you need more of it? (Spoiler alert: personally, I reckon we can all lean more toward the latter.)

THE POSTMODERN FITLOSOPHER

I'm about to frustrate and vex your wonderful brains, dear reader: in truth, postmodernism has yet to be pinned down with one definitive framework to follow. That postmodernism is technically indefinable is not an incorrect assumption. When we describe postmodernism, we refer to a set of rhetoric that criticises current frameworks and definitions, including epistemology or how we perceive the world around us.

Postmodernism is a funny concept and one that is a bit tricky to describe, even in a longer format such as this one. It first entered the trajectory of philosophical debate in the 1970s. For one philosopher, Jean Francois-Lyotard, postmodernism was to become a rejection of meta-narratives to be skeptical of frameworks that emancipate ourselves from the structures we reside in. It is a critique of modernist concepts, which is already problematic in the way we systemise it as a philosophy, partly due to linguistic and cultural differences. For instance, the modernist movement in Portugal was galvanised in the '60s, inspired and based by the fascination surrounding aesthetics and narrative founded in Italy about a decade prior. This form of modernism cared not for revolution but of historical analysis and engagement in the arts. The Italian form of postmodernism bases itself on discussing society's narrative and continuity issues rather than counteracting against the ideals heralded prior to modernism.

> "Lamenting the 'loss of meaning' in postmodernity boils down to mourning the fact that knowledge is no longer principally narrative" (Lyotard 1984 [1979], 26). Here, Lyotard comments on the fact that our dissemination of knowledge into information (which are distinct concepts, in philosophy at least) has meant that language and transferal of thoughts and ideas are now too heterogeneous—in other words, disparate—to create a coherent identity or truth. This feeds into the idea amongst most postmodern thinkers that there is no real, solidified "truth."

Yet, for the French, modernism was very much a structuralist concept, conversing with concepts like Marxism in an attempt to discuss the gaps and debate surrounding sociocultural progress. In essence, postmodernism is not necessarily an attack on modernism (though granted, they must engage with, and at times, criticise the material preceding it) but more of a proposed approach as to how we can understand contemporary thinking and apply it to the way we live.

Deconstruction is a popular term often banded about alongside postmodernism, and in some ways, you'd be right to interweave the two of them at times. However, in philosophy, there is actually a concrete definition we can use to systemise it. Deconstruction alludes to applying certain techniques for reading and interpreting various texts. The term was introduced into philosophical literature in 1967 by Jacques Derrida, who, despite insisting a separation from postmodernism overall, is generally associated with the latter movement due to his contributions toward truth and knowledge. Derrida famously once said that there is no "outside text"; in other words, due to the various language games and technical progress from modernist thinking, function has overwritten metaphysics, and consequently, universal truth eludes us. He has become quite a controversial figure for both the left and right in politics, assumedly a figure of relativism and nihilism. While it is tempting to assume such a notion, his thoughts on modernist development promote lateral, critical thinking and exertion of skepticism over entrenched, traditional rituals.

As we can see just from this tiny, meagre summary of the movement, a plethora of issues raises its head when it comes to pinning down its aims and values. First, the term itself is pretty vague. Postmodernism is used to refer to a bunch of groups doing all sorts of different things with varying agendas. There is very little in common, for instance, between Kurt Vonnegut and Jacques Derrida, yet they are both considered "postmodern" in their approaches.

Second, people are confused about what is in the movement. Some, for instance, mistake Marxism or surrealism as being part of it, despite the fact that those are actually modernist movements; Marxism is an example of the kind of political theory that is most often the target of postmodernist critique, after all, as it is considered a meta-narrative to be scorned at. And don't get me started on the notion of "neo marxism;" this concept is a term respected neither within the realm of philosophy nor outside of it.

Okay, great. Now my brain hurts. What's the deal if I'm a Postmodernist Fitlosopher? Do I believe in truth?

This is a great deal of information to chew over, and it can feel particularly frustrating when the endgame of a philosophical concept is, simply put, to explore and question rather than have a set of concrete values and ideas as seen in previous chapters. Instead, postmodernism offers us freedom in many forms of discipline, characterised by skepticism and debate. In a way, for the Postmodernist Fitlosopher, this notion offers us malleability and adaptability in the way we train and create a lifestyle.

As implicated from its philosophical counterpart, a Postmodernist Fitlosopher might exude a natural skepticism toward the traditional, tried-and-tested rituals peppered within the fitness industry, adopting instead an open and curious approach to training and nutrition.

You might consider yourself to be a Postmodernist Fitlosopher if you find yourself uttering similar sentiments to these:

1. "There's no one-size-fits-all when it comes to training and nutrition. Universal truth doesn't exist."
2. "Technically, there's no such thing as a barbell: there's more than one way to create resistance and muscle growth. There's no definitive direction for strength gain."
3. "Calories are a social construct, and henceforth I shall be disbanding them." (Naturally, the last statement is tongue-in-cheek—do not recommend clinging to that aphorism like fur to a cat!)

There's a massive advantage to encouraging a skeptical, flowing stream of consciousness when it comes to cultivating your own lifestyle. For one, you're more likely to disengage with current fitness commentaries, such as cultural tropes regarding bodyweight and moral value. A Postmodernist Fitlosopher will be excellent at deconstructing (ha, see what I did there?) the logical and moral failings implicated with associating aesthetics and appearance with one's own sense of worth.

Taking a postmodernist argument, for instance, the concept of weight loss is an invariable, sole route of lifestyle change is void because there would be, in the eyes of a Postmodernist Fitlosopher, no universal truth in how we approach a goal. Indeed, the theories underlined by hosts of strength and conditioning coaches mirror Hegelian and Marxist models of thought in that they believe there is a constant back and forth of discussion within the industry to further coaching and thought in order to "perfect" the art of personal training.

You see this same idea within Marx and Hegel's proposal that history unravels itself through a consistent back-and-forth of events and class differences, essentially creating what we know to be a synthesis of the material conditions at any given time. This, in theory, progresses society. Similarly, this line of thought would be analogous to conversations in the fitness industry regarding approaches to calorie deficits or training reaching a "pinnacle," or progression of the art itself.

Postmodernist Fitlosophers would be inclined to disagree. Much like postmodernist thinkers like Lyotard believed the language to be too disparate to create a united framework of sociocultural definitions, Postmodernist Fitlosophers may also argue that there is no one set approach in either coaching or choosing one's own lifestyle adjustments.

And, in truth, they'd be right. Now more than ever, we are realising that health is much, much more than just a number on the scale. A number of factors dovetail with one another but in the sense of causation and consequence. These factors may range from the purely biomedical—our genes, neurobiology, and bio-mechanics—to the downright social—economic status, upbring-ing, and worldview. The reason for this relies upon an emerging branch of research known as epigenetics. Epigenetics essentially encompasses a biopsychosocial approach in that it incorporates all three models of health to understand our well-being and lifestyle factors. Epigenetics literally means "beyond genetics," and as the phrase suggests, it tries to explain how our genes and chromo-somes express ourselves in light of environmental stimuli.

This seems complicated, and it is. Without going too far into the science and potentially boring you, epigenetics involves genes "turning on or off" based upon a person's environmental circum-stances. For instance, in theory, epigenetics would suggest that depression is hereditary, which means that you don't just magically get low episodes because of your ingrained biology, but rather that you might have the proclivity to, based on your environment and genetic structure interplaying with one another.

Person A might have one gene that predisposes them to certain vulnerabilities, be it a mental illness or physical ailment. Person B does not have said gene. Throw both people into the same stressful scenario, for instance, getting an undesired grade or losing employment, and according to epigenetic theory, they'll both react differently despite this same expression of circumstance. Person A's gene "switches on" as a result of the level of stress and puts them in a more vulnerable position to become depressed or anxious, whereas Person B has no such gene to express these ailments.

What has this got to do with postmodernism, one may ask, especially as I'm attempting to use scientific research, a concept fairly scorned by some postmodernists, to buttress my point? Simply put, the nascence of epigenetics exposes the vulnerability of science and how one day we can be right, and in one fell swoop, totally off the mark. This perfectly encapsulates postmodernism's emphasis that the worship on such a heterogenous framework leads to no consolidation of ideas.

This absolutely does not mean a dismissal of science, rather an exploration of what these ideas mean to us, and how we can make sense of them in our culture overall.

Postmodernist Fitlosophers, as a result, may argue that the scientific consensus on calories in, calories out is pointless without a decided-upon construct for each individual. Things like cultural pressures to conform or look or train a certain way are eschewed, as they are mere constructs to be taken apart and debated. Instead, Postmodernist Fitlosophers will likely question the status quo and conclude thus: fitness and health are extremely individual, offering freedom from external pressures or obligations to perform in a certain vein. They are liberated from the binds of societal expectations and constructed tropes.

What's so good about being "free"?

With malleability comes creativity, first and foremost. Postmodernists overall in thought will be more interested in the vacuum between the signifier and the signified; that is, they are preoccupied with meaning-making, rather than the meaning behind something itself—how things mean rather than what they mean.

Likely to have a sharp and curious mind, Postmodernist Fitlosophers will have accrued this sense of meaning-making in the way they interpret a fitness goal. For instance, they'll understand that progressive overload—the act of getting stronger via creating gradual adaptations in their training—is not merely limited to the act of lifting a barbell. It can look like many things: manipulation of force via ground reaction, the momentum of their own body weight, or tweaking of tempo, for example. They are more likely to add variability and variety into their training as opposed to strictly adhering to traditional concepts.

Likewise, they might see the act of calorie tracking as a form of social inertia as sorts. A Postmodernist Fitlosopher might be more likely to eat intuitively. In this piece, we will define intuitive eating as the concept of listening to your own internal and external needs rather than abiding by an app or dietary goal. Neither approach is inherently wrong, it must be noted. But a Postmodernist Fitlosopher will be defiant of fitness group norms and conform to the beat of their own drum by engaging with the cultural tropes at hand.

In essence, there's much good to be had at adopting openness in overall lifestyle change. It allows one peace of mind; a person is much less likely to suffer from low self-esteem, anxiety, and even loneliness when cultivating their own mind and voice on approaches. Having a degree of skepticism toward current industry structures might be useful in encouraging this way of thinking.

Postmodernist Fitlosophers will scorn standardised norms in favour of thinking for themselves and what works best for their lives. They head toward their goals with an emboldened sense of what's right and wrong for their goals and an ability to critically think, carving out a more wholesome and inclusive narrative for the industry as a whole.

Postmodernist Fitlosophers might be more inclined to challenge the following narratives which permeate the fitness sociocultural system:

1. **The notion that weight purely predicates health.** Whilst we do have absolute, statistical measurements implicating body mass with certain conditions, it truly is just that—an implication. Health is a complex faction, and an individual's weight is just one piece of the pie, pun not intended. A Postmodernist Fitlosopher will happily call out the biomedical, reductionist lens of examining health purely by the metrics of a scale number.

2. **Defying ensconced, entrenched attitudes and norms.** A Postmodernist Fitlosopher will express concern for the norms permeated and entrenched within the industry itself. They'll be much more adept at challenging these frameworks due to the dissolution of one universal "truth" as perpetrated by the postmodernist movement.

These traits of societal critique are admirable. Yet, some issues remain if we delve too far into the realm of postmodernist thought. These gaps in the argument of postmodernist thought have permeated dialogue for decades, and unfortunately, we're going to have to do the same when it comes to something as microcosmic as a lifestyle change.

Can it just become a free-for-all?

Postmodernism faces problems a priori due to its unstable definitions, fluctuating without much warning between thinkers and generations. Materialist philosophers in contemporary settings have accused postmodernism of failing to deconstruct the very modernist matrix they claim to break down (things like subject or nature or culture, for instance). In fact, it might be proposed that postmodernism actually reifies the constraints it seeks to unravel. Claims about diet culture, for example, runs the risk of creating a culture within itself, which leads to an **invalid and unsound** argument or premise.

Postmodernism purports to be post-ideological and maintains a disdain of meta-narratives, like science or philosophy or a specific type of aesthetic. You know how when people say that philosophy is pointless, that they actually ironically end up stating something utilising philosophy? A very similar thing occurs in the fallout of postmodernist arguments. The hyper-focus on ideology and meta-narrative is a massive *example of* ideology or meta-narrative insofar as it casts itself beyond such things only to judge all others based on its own premise.

As such, the extreme subjectivity postmodernism exerts ends up actually *dismantling* subjectivity. So a major problem that lies within postmodernism is that there's very little to actually critique using its lens since its position as a movement is partially the absence of a position of any "truth."

Modernism was a movement driven by questioning, whereas postmodernism is associated with flat-out denial.

Hence, people have become increasingly skeptical of postmodernism's claims. Such demand for subjectivity can prove problematic when trying to investigate empirical issues. The latter is important when we consider cultivating an evidence-based lifestyle change.

Postmodernist Fitlosophers might indeed have a proclivity toward openness, creativity, and questioning societal norms, but all of this can venture too far into the realms of science denial if not careful. Consider for a moment the current polemic surrounding diet culture. There are undoubtedly discussions to be had surrounding societal tropes encouraging us to conform to set standards or ideals and the impact these facets may have on our overall mental well-being and self-image. Nonetheless, to ignore the biological is a rookie error, simply put.

Intuitive eating, for example, is often purported to be a simple solution to the calorie-counting alternative. Yet research suggests that it is an art to be practiced. It is not, as the name suggests, something that comes to us freely. "Intuitive" is a misnomer; indeed, one can demand chocolate or doughnuts simply by listening to the gentle, spontaneous whim that emerges in our brain. Restriction and self-flagellation certainly isn't the answer, but neither is assuming that every demand is one to be satisfied. The research behind intuitive eating, as an example, actually implies that in order to be skilled at such a habit, one needs knowledge a priori of what they eat and how they feel as a consequence. The sense of tracking—or, at least, semi-awareness—of what one consumes is implicit in the act.

This is just an example of how a postmodernist argument can hamper even the most well-intentioned of deconstructivism attempts. If a Postmodernist Fitlosopher finds themselves feeling listless or lacking concrete goals, it might behoove them to step back and appreciate the empirical nature required for changes in nutrition or training.

Asking themselves questions, like:

1. How consistent is my argument with my original premise?
2. If I say that A is B, and B is C, can I really conclude that A can also be D, E, or F?
3. What are the other arguments supporting my/other suppositions?

This is not to say that their social critique is wrong. Indeed, those who fall into the lens of a Marxist Fitlosopher may lean too far the other way and require this openness and subjectivity that enables a different kind of thinking. But sometimes, Postmodernist Fitlosophers may benefit greatly from structure, framework, and rules that supplant their critique with a stronger argument whilst honouring the validity of the scientific method laid out today.

THE UTILITARIAN FITLOSOPHER

Believe it or not, moral dilemmas make for excellent storytelling. One way or another, we are compelled by the reasons why an individual in a film or book does the things they do. Take Batman, for instance; in Christopher Nolan's critically acclaimed work *The Dark Knight*, our caped crusader has an opportunity to kill his formidable nemesis, the Joker, before the latter escapes the hubbub and splendour of Bruce Wayne's penthouse party. This all comes at the cost of allowing love-interest Rachel Dawes to hurtle downward to inevitable death from said rooftop. Naturally, Bruce Wayne's instinctive reaction is to chase after the woman he loves. On top of that, Batman boasts a simple yet measurable doctrine in his crime-fighting undertakings: never kill, no matter the crime. Yet some philosophers, were they to watch this very scene, might have a curmudgeonly response to this intuition.

Indeed, if each of us were to plop onto our heads a miserly philosopher hat, we could formulate the case that Batman's decision stemmed from emotion and compulsion. The Joker is an undisputed threat to society, in existential and practical terms; at that point in time of the story, he had killed many people and would have gone onto murder many more innocent civilians. In short, there might be less societal unhappiness if a criminal like the Joker were to be eradicated from existence. The philosophy that strives for the action that leads to the greatest amount of happiness for the greatest number of people is known as **utilitarianism**. Utilitarianism is a school of thought oft attributed to many thinkers throughout the ages. So, it'd feel inane to go into excessive individual detail here when we're simply grappling with behavioural approaches to lifestyle change. There are a few Classical Utilitarians—those who championed this famed approach to normative ethics—who are worth knowing about: Jeremy Bentham and John Stuart Mill. Bentham liked to think about the way we behaved in terms of social utility. That is to say, we as human beings naturally seek out outcomes that promulgate happiness. Naturally, this in part implies we avoid painful or harm-provoking tools of action.

Inspired by the trailblazers that set alight the intellectual path before his time, Bentham took the notions set forth by the Enlightenment and sought to create an empirical overview of human nature. Quite the task if you ask anyone. In short, Bentham attempted to "calculate" what it meant for an individual to be happy. He came to the conclusion that happiness could be attained by experiencing a lack of pain and indirectly maximising one's personal pleasure. If it was a math equation, you'd be adding up all the good stuff but subtracting the things that dampen your well-being. What was a revolutionary turn in moral, normative ethics appears practical to us; rather than viewing actions as inherently "wrong" based on a prescribed moral label (Kantian ethics tends to lean into this), Bentham tried to extrapolate the good and bad in actions through their utility. Thus we produce the aptly-named moniker of philosophical thought. Utilitarianism is considered a form of consequentialism; as the name suggests, it espouses an emphasis on the outcome of an action. You could make the case that including a notion of utility spices things up a bit in the normative ethics bedroom. Utilitarianism considered everyone's interests equally, not solely the consequences of a given outcome in and of itself.

Already, there should be some pink-tinted flags being raised in the direction of anybody wanting to make lifestyle changes. If Bentham assumes happiness to be quantitative (which he does), that means we can't create a descriptive framework in which to specify what pleasure is and isn't. That means scoffing a box of Krispy Kreme or forgoing a daily walk for Netflix binges could be considered acts of minimising one's pain and thus maximising happiness. In truth, we know that these habits might tickle that dopaminergic itch in a fleeting instance, but to suggest they evoke long-term fulfillment or happiness is a bit of a stretch. This could be interpreted as a flaw in a Utilitarian Fitlosopher's line of behaving. If it feels good, it must be destined for my greater happiness, right? Unfortunately, if that were true, things that made us feel good all the time would lead to success, and hardship and pain would dissipate from society's collective ethos entirely. There must've been a way to rectify Bentham's loophole, then, if utilitarianism was to become as popular an ethical approach as it has done. Cue John Stuart Mill, who endeavoured to address this logical inconsistency with aplomb in his aptly named essay, "Utilitarianism."

John Stuart Mill saw what Bentham did and liked it. Though, like any good philosopher, he couldn't help but nitpick. After all, if you don't create some form of minor contention or arbitrary, asinine nitpicking of a predecessor's argument, are you even philosophising? The answer, of course, is a resounding no. Mill saw the problem with equating all forms of pleasure with happiness—the same way we just did with a standardised Utilitarian Fitlosophy approach—and sought to counter these intuitions against certain types of pleasure. Notably, we could consider Mill to be a bit more specific in the way he views happiness and pleasure compared to Bentham. He noted that certain activities—reading a book, taking a stroll through the park, or sharing a social communion with loved ones, as examples—carried more weight and meaning than the hedonism we usually associate with gratification. We don't have to confine our philosophical analogies to Batman's (anti)heroics. It can be just as, if not more, practical and informative to apply utilitarianism as a way of moderating our indulgences. If Bentham ranked all forms of pleasure-seeking as a means of invoking happiness, the logic follows that he'd assume scoffing an extra-large pizza in front of the television to be on the same level of meaning as writing a beautiful poem or solving a complex physics equation. Our intuitions know this to feel jarring.

In the same vein, can we really consider hitting a weight-lifting personal best to evoke the same "sensation" of happiness as drinking a beer on the couch? Whether you're a philosopher or not, the answer is clearly no. That's not to label the latter as immoral or bad. However, what it does do is distinguish between different types of happiness and pleasure. Mill was keen on doing this so as not to conflate utilitarianism as a free-for-all, to do with whatever one pleases at any given time. A Utilitarian Fitlosopher is (hopefully) sensible enough to intuit this; they'll be an individual who lives vicariously through Mill's assertion that happiness is "a good" people will aim to attain for. There's an implication here, suggesting what "should" be desired. A Utilitarian Fitlosopher might strive for happiness in many ways. For some, understanding happiness might involve recognising the joys of moderation and fitting in foods they enjoy within their energy intake, rather than opting for dietary self-flagellation.

Where have I seen this word before?

You might see many science-minded individuals espouse, knowingly or not, concepts that are rooted within the school of utilitarianism. This is because the very nature of utilitarianism is based upon empirical investigation. In other words, it tries to "calculate" morality, or how we should behave, in ways that are measurable and verifiable. Naturally, this is in keeping with the structure of the scientific method: propose hypotheses and search for a way to disprove them.

Never has an example of utilitarianism been so prevalently used in contemporary dialogue more so than the COVID-19 pandemic. The constant dialogue or "weighing up" between loss of life via virus or lockdown is an instance of scientists and politicians attempting to find a "greater good" in the midst of chaos. Indeed, it proved to be a kind of trolley problem in real-time.

In any case, try and spot pragmatic uses of this ethical approach in daily living. It could be as simple as your manager picking a different spot for the team lunch based on the group's overall preferences and needs over their own. Once you identify this, you'll be able to pinpoint aspects of personal utilitarianism in your lifestyle adaptations. Do you pick the pizza or the protein bar? Which one offers greater levels of happiness (as per outlined by Mill) than the other? There is no wrong answer. The response will differ from person to person, depending on where we are in our own personal journeys.

The (empirically driven, philosophically sound) Pursuit of Happiness?

This section has given us a basic idea of how Bentham and Mill thought we could tackle moral and ethical quandaries. Within that idea, a framework is born: a type of personalised set of scales, so attuned to our human follies and desires they'd make Lady Justice blush with envy. In all the things we do, we might find ourselves weighing up the decisions to lead to a contented day. Do we lie in and catch up on sleep, or get up early to finish a dastardly report? Will going to the gym give us the same boost of dopaminergic joy we find in beloved Netflix specials? If you find yourself making lifestyle-based decisions orientated around this process of elimination, you might be a natural Utilitarian Fitlosopher.

Utilitarian Fitlosophers have the possibility of falling into different camps in similar ways to how Bentham and Mills interpreted happiness differently. Sure, it's entirely possible to view self-indulgence as the same thing as long-term happiness—it is, after all, numbing any potential pain receptors, in both a holistic and neurobiological sense—but your typical Utilitarian Fitlosopher will err on the side of Mills, here's hoping. There'll be an appreciation that what you do now affects your tomorrow. In other words, removal of one's pain—or increasing base levels of happiness—cannot be equated to eating whatever the hell you want or avoiding the discomfort of an early morning workout. It is more painful, arguably so, to be stuck in the same place you were a day, week, month, or even a year ago. The Utilitarian Fitlosopher might equate this kind of pain with being more severe and psychologically taxing than the discomfort of altering lifestyle habits for improved performance. This is a very Mills-esque way of viewing overarching health and well-being.

So can the Utilitarian Fitlosopher quantify such a thing as happiness? I mean, ask most psychologists, and they'll reply that there're a few mechanisms of measuring specific metrics, even if they're self-reported. Research often takes into account certain kinds of questionnaires, which attempt to reveal maladaptive behaviours or thought patterns among individuals. We can only hazard a well-educated guess, but from that basis, we can conclude whether a person is adopting a higher-level quality of life compared to another. Based on this, a Utilitarian Fitlosopher's pursuit of happiness might be founded upon their own bespoke framework. Billy the Powerlifter will examine his routine and argue that lifting heavy tin four times a week and schlepping down protein shakes is a superior approach to keeping himself ticking over. On the other hand, busy mum Sarah sees cutting down her wine intake from two glasses a night to one—and squeezing in the odd walk—as the ideal methods of "reducing" her perceived pain. If she tied to follow Billy the Powerlifter's regime, she'd be miserable; it's not as simple as assuming more exercise, more protein equates to alleviating stress levels. To maximise Sarah's happiness, we have to look at her life in an overarching fashion: how will she spend time with her kids? Find time for her partner? Put food on the table whilst juggling it all? Her "equation" to reducing stress and pain will not look the same as an elite athlete's formula. In fact, giving her the same health blueprint as Billy will most certainly exaggerate her pain rather than reduce it.

Odds are the Utilitarian Fitlosopher is particularly apt at understanding this. Yet there runs the risk of twisting and misinterpreting what it means to be happy, what it means to moderate pain and stress levels. Aphorisms like "self-care" can be seen as doing whatever feels good in a given time or a spontaneous instance. Pizza and chocolate certainly help us feel better momentarily, but whether the consistent overindulgence in these types of foods leads to a Mills-type of happiness is up for debate. That said, we absolutely need to separate overtly conservative views on food. Terms such as "cheat meals" take away our agency as adults; we base our happiness or settle our woes with meals that rival the splendour of Henry VIII's banquets, then get into a cycle of self-hatred and guilt over a conglomerate of carbohydrates and fats. Humans truly do the best they can at infuriating themselves and others.

Happiness in this sense cannot be accounted for solely by the greenery on your plate or the macro balance popping out from your My Fitness Pal app. It is more holistic than that. Throughout history, we've honoured our relations both with ourselves and to others through the act of eating and food preparation. There are resolute, neuropsychological benefits to enjoying a moderate lifestyle, as it enables us to incorporate psychological flexibility and explore who we are as fully fledged whole beings. An example of this would be managing anxiety around food or social events. Incorporating moderation as a means of lifestyle change would result in regulating our nervous systems, meaning we're less likely to feel overly stressed about dietary choices or spending time with loved ones without a Tupperware box. That "on edge" feeling one gets, like floaty butterflies in the stomach or a racing heart, can be endemic of this shift into stressing and nervousness. Naturally, there's a much lesser chance of developing rigid tendencies with food or even anxiety-induced disorders. If we rigidly adhere to just one level of living, we deny who we are as humans. Even top-tier athletes schedule downtime relative to their hefty training schedules.

Utilitarian Fitlosophers are likely to look at the bigger picture to see the "greater good" in terms of what will benefit them and their lives overall. Sometimes that might be a pizza, and other times, it's getting up early in the morning to squeeze in their training.

There's a mechanical, formulaic way in how they view their goals and habits. In this sense, they become individuals who have a solid grasp of what they value and the longstanding actions required to achieve these motivational drivers. This provides an excellent basis for any type of behavioural change; utilitarianism helps sort out the practical wheat from the chaff, in some sense.

Miscalculations—and Human Error

Still, what about Rachael Dawes?

If utilitarianism is indeed about calculating some sort of optimal outcome, it begs the question: how can we focus primarily on the outcome without negating the process itself?

In the case of Batman killing Joker rather than saving Rachael, the utilitarian would argue that the outcome of Joker being dead outweighed the action of saving another human being. The good of the many, they might argue, is a priority over the life of one innocent. If this feels somewhat disparaging, that's natural: the ethical implications of ignoring action over outcome—which, let's face it, is unpredictable in any case—is a famed critique of utilitarian philosophy.

So, two issues lay ahead of us here: one, that negating all actions over the outcome, such as letting an innocent woman die in favour of an outcome that might not even happen, and two, that we cannot predict any set given circumstance to unfold as our utilitarian "calculations" might foretell. In other words, twenty-year-old you is different than thirty-year-old you. If you try and make decisions solely based on what thirty-year-old you might prefer now, there's no guarantee these outcomes will benefit you as you once thought.

Philosophers might spend lengthy amounts of time attempting to compute these outcomes, but at the end of the day, they are still human. And humans make mistakes.

A Utilitarian Fitlosopher can only act based upon *potential* predictions about *potential* versions of themselves. They cannot guarantee that the energy they pour into a specific goal now will be relevant in a year's time, say—or perhaps even less than that. This is one of the reasons we mere mortals revere and respect the routine of higher-tier athletes so much: in spite of life's uncertain maelstrom, both internal and external, they have a game plan, and they stick to it.

So a Utilitarian Fitlosopher might base their "greater good" upon a concept that in years to come means nothing to them. That's not to say their efforts would be worthless in that scenario; indeed, nothing can be nobler than having a meaningful pursuit, even if your values or motivations shift over time. The emphasis on outcome might be problematic too; if an individual finds that their social or personal life is suffering at the hands of the "greater good" of meal prep, weight loss goals, or even sporting performance (unless, of course, the latter is quite literally what is paying their rent), their psychological flexibility may diminish. Exerting excessive stringency toward an outcome—an outcome which, by the way, we cannot truly calculate for—can lead to individuals fostering an insular attitude as much as a Kantian approach could instigate. When we consider the potential triggers for higher stress levels or even bouts of loneliness or depression in contemporary society, we cannot neglect the fact that food is interwoven into our sociocultural tapestry. The "greater good" isn't so great if we don't adapt to potential errors.

There's also the issue of how one even begins to interpret happiness. As we've seen from Bentham and Mill's approaches, happiness is a subjective moniker that ducks and weaves in a non-linear fashion over time. In our relationships with friends, family, and significant others, for example, I dare you to claim that you feel ardent bliss at all times of the day, every day. If that's the case, then you're probably interacting with a bespoke-made robot, not a human being. I'd argue there are days that any given relationship might actually bring you stress or even pain at that moment. Yet does that detract from its meaning and value in our lives? We cannot use formulae or constructs to discern what can or will make us happy at any given time. The Utilitarian Fitlosopher, in short, might try to calculate the incalculable, measure the immeasurable.

Moral Snake-Eating

There is a funny kind of irony in the contrasts between utilitarianism and deontology. Despite Mills and Kant offering very different models of ethics, both end up eating the tail of the snake when it comes to Fitlosophy.

Utilitarian Fitlosophers try to calculate happiness or predict how x will affect y in any given space in time, whilst Kantian Fitlosophers propose the notion of objective morality, and therefore, a concretely right and wrong way to live. Both of these have their merits in cultivating discipline and routine for an individual's life. Nonetheless, both categories of Fitlosophers require a loosening of frameworks, understanding that sometimes, life—and indeed, the follies of human beings—can not always confer to the stern words of wisened philosophy. They provide excellent metrics to help us become the people we want to be, certainly. But if you find that you're stuck to this notion of "greater good" and not necessarily taking the time out of your day to see the good that's right out there in front of you, it may serve you well to take a step back and look at more fluid interpretations of the world. The previous chapter's take on the Postmodernist Fitlosopher is a decent example of implementing this level of psychological flexibility.

In a world of incalculable and—yes, pardon the now-frivolous use of the term—unprecedented times, there can be solace in how we try and predict outcomes or formulate some kind of solution for life's tumultuousness. Having said that, there's also a beauty in letting go of any given certainty. Injuries happen. Perhaps you get sick and nutritional needs to change. Maybe you fall in love with a sport and find one way of "doing fitness" no longer serves your goals. In any case, the Utilitarian Fitlosopher may need to find a way of reconciling this unpredictability with their precise calculations. The only outcome we can predict in life, after all, is the certainty that change can and will occur.

IMMANUEL KANT AND THE KANTIAN FITLOSOPHER

Odds are, if you ask someone to name a philosopher that they "know," however vaguely or obtusely, Immanuel Kant's title will probably pop up alongside the ancient greats. Whether you think he's a wisdom-imbued genius or a total bore who grew old before his time, Kant's contributions to philosophy have stood the test of time, namely for their practical applications easily viewed in our contemporary times.

Kant is often the guy that gets the most flack at schmoozy dinner parties or intellectual discussions. A particularly prominent feature in the intelligentsia of today, after all, is the notion of **relativism**. This is a funny little concept which, as previously mentioned, declares that there is no solidified theory of objective morality or set of ethics. One may even wonder if, should we go down the rabbit hole deep enough we become guilty of dismissing claims that we should, well, care for anything at all.

Ironically, the quandary of whether or not we should even care at all is a primer of moral philosophy. When you ponder upon vastly profound notions like, "Why should we care?" or "What's the big deal?" you're essentially questioning the value of something. Is it worth our time and attention? Is it better or worse than something else? If it's a question of value, then—ding, ding, ding, you guessed it—they all fall under the umbrella of moral philosophy.

I'm guessing, nay, hoping that swathes of you haven't just read the term moral philosophy and instead gone onto your phones to scroll through a variety of meme pages. If that's the case, you must be a serious masochist for getting this far through *Fitlosophy*. Kudos to you.

Even those who espouse relativist values are signposting themselves to a position of values and judgment-based statements, even if they're not aware of it. A statement declaring that something has little to no meaning is in itself a proposal that carries actual meaning.

I know this is a bit of a headache but do your best to hang in there with me.

Kant looked at this relativist stance on morality and had none of it. He proposed the idea that any potential ethical framework put forward had to be consistently "right" or "wrong" in all scenarios. That means that lying to your partner, saying they look good in their dress when in your mind, Beetlejuice's pinstriped, dirt-caked suit looked more flattering, is wrong in the eyes of Kant. No matter how much said-partner might fawn and coo over your fluffy soufflé of niceness that coats your words.

Like any philosopher, of course, his arguments have their share of inconsistencies (seeking the truth and thinking for yourself is the beauty of philosophy, in any case), and yet his categorical imperative remains one of the more popular ways of viewing morality within its lens. A Kantian Fitlosopher, no doubt, would share his emphasis on the importance of duty-based morality and leading a life that involves a regimen with lists of conditions longer than a Leonard Cohen song. Kant's school of philosophy is known as **deontology**, but for the sake of consistency and ease in this part of the series, we'll simply be referring to his namesake when discussing his ideas.

Kant's philosophy revolves around universals, as the categorical imperative suggests.

It's entirely facile for us contemporaneous readers to guffaw at his rigid routine that aged him more than a dodgy sunbed tan. But there's no denying his contributions to philosophy have, and remain to be, some of the most important fundamentals in philosophical thinking, particularly those pertaining to ethics. He wanted to create a universality to morality in that he proposed there could be a codified set of ethics that applied to all humans, all the time, everywhere. Granted, this theory has been rebuked countless times by other philosophers, both past and present, but several edifices of his thinking have still stood the test of time, nonetheless.

According to Kant, some actions were to be considered prohibited—his views on lying generally fall under this category, for instance. Said actions, even if they increased maximal happiness, could only be depended upon if they fulfilled our moral duties or not. This is essentially a huge 180 from the previously discussed Utilitarian philosophy.

For Kant, being human meant being something special and not in the casual use which we are typically used to. Kant believed our consciousness was sacred. In other words, our rational faculties, ability to decipher right from wrong and navigate ourselves around the clusterfuckery that is our society. Creatures or inanimate objects, says Kant, do not boast such an ability. Thus, we create a sort of special moral sphere wherein our capacity to reason and experience consciousness creates a necessary framework to behave in a set way. In other words, it is due to our humanity that we are due to follow an objective morality as part of our duty to the society around us.

I mean, what kind of "duty" can we even fulfill when we're trying to eat a bit better or move around more?

Kantian Fitlosophers, as a result, may fall into similarly duty-based procedures when it comes to starting a new routine or embarking upon habit change. One of the most admirable traits of their working model is their commitment to said changes and stalwart refusal to backtrack or tweak, even if they find it difficult. Moreover, as they recognise the importance of following their own system of values, habit change becomes a great deal more pleasurable—in the most Kantian sense of the term, of course. Kantian Fitlosophers are able to discern between that instantaneous buzz of several doughnuts or a Netflix binge session and instead heed the fact that long-term contentment and meaning is the driving goal, not short-term pleasantries.

A Kantian Fitlosopher may be more likely to view their lifestyle change as something akin to being dutiful toward others. And this likely means not using people as means to something. Instead, they consider their actions carefully, thinking about whether or not they train or eat well has more nefarious ends rather than duty-based ones.

What do we mean when we discuss means and ends? When we consider our actions in general, we think about the end results of why we do a certain something. For example, if I feel hungry, I'll likely go to the kitchen and pour myself a bowl of Rice Krispies because 1) cereal for dinner when in adulthood is severely underrated and 2) I want to fill the gaping hole in my stomach (and possibly heart.) The cereal in this case is the end goal, as it helps me assuage my hunger and crack on with my day. I might feel a bit too lazy to get into the kitchen and undergo the arduous, gargantuan task of filling up my cereal bowl, but it is necessary means to reach said-end of eating the cereal. A means is how we get to our specific end, and an end is something that is desired for its own sake.

Let's take another example whereby Kant might argue our means and ends get muddled ever so slightly. Let's say I want to get healthy, and so I take up a certain exercise routine or change my diet in order to do so. The end in this case might be to get healthy, and the means would be the mentioned activities taken to get there. A mean is a thing we might do conditionally—it's not that we exactly want to get up and go to the gym at five in the morning, but given busy timetables conflicting with our desired goal, it may be the only way to get to the end of improved health. That end could be extended even further, and the means become a barometer for something much more, something deeply entrenched. It may appear that I attend to these means for the end of getting healthier, but really, it might be that I want to fit into my old dress to appear more attractive or feel confident in myself or feel like I can prove to others that I can stick to a weight loss program. In which case, the end has changed significantly. Whilst this in of itself is no bad thing, Kant demanded that we treated neither ourselves nor others as a means to an end. A Kantian Fitlosopher will therefore analyse the reasons behind the actions preceding his goals and checking to see whether or not they align with their overall values or are a fleeting panacea to tend to a greater wound.

In essence: our means to intended ends, and the ends themselves, matter according to Kant. This means a Kantian Fitlosopher is likely to be prudent and pragmatic in outlining or identifying their northern star.

Kantian Fitlosophers may ask themselves the following before deciding upon an action to take:

(i) Can I rationally will that everyone act as I propose to act? (In other words, would you like others to follow your proposed moral framework?) If the answer is no, then we must not perform the action.

(ii) *Does my action respect the goals of human beings rather than merely using them for my own purposes? Again, if the answer is no, then we must not perform the action. (Kant believed that these questions were equivalent.)*

Man, I Kant believe he was such a stickler for rules.

Is there any moral obligation to improve oneself, to foster and develop various capacities in oneself? From a broadly Kantian point of view, self-improvement defends the view that there is such an obligation and that it is an obligation that each person owes to him or herself.

This also ties in with *ii*, from above. When we are able to maximise our own well-being and health, we can become better friends, sisters, brothers, sons, or daughters. We are able to fulfill our potential as contributing, kind members of society and add meaning not only to our own lives but to others' experiences as well.

A Kantian Fitlosopher may not necessarily turn their nose up toward externally driven sources of motivation. We are, after all, only human and are unable to fully escape from the evolutionary desire to walk down the street with lingering eyes, potentially un-dressing us mentally until we catch a chill. The issue is whether that becomes our sole end. Are we solely trying to gain validation from others for sex, social status, even self-validation? Or is there a somewhat greater end? What would that attraction represent? Would it negate years of negative self-talk, poor mental health issues, or defiance of stringent, conservative doctrines that have prevented them from exploring this side of dating?

All to say, a Kantian's take on means and ends can result in fruitful exploration of our true desires. A Kantian Fitlosopher may hope to carve out nobler goals than a twelve-week transformation, which relies purely on physical matters and corporeal concerns.

And, as argued by Kant, if there were no duties to oneself, then "there would be no duties whatsoever." In other words, if we can-not apply the level of self-care and respect to ourselves, then it could prove difficult to assign it across the board to loved ones or even wider society.

Therefore, if we define health and fitness as a form of self-care and an extension of self-development, then we can identify it as a necessary duty to fulfill in order to fulfill *ii*.

Because it abides by our sense of duty, it extends to improving others' lives, and therefore benefiting society as a whole rather than just our individual selves.

By seeing fitness as something less intrinsically selfish, and something that can actually create a "domino effect" of positive change across the board, then we are more than likely maximising our adherence to a healthy routine and reaching our fitness goals. As motivation is intrinsic rather than extrinsic, we tend to see the pro-cess of improving our fitness as something more enriching and not just a superficial pursuit. It is when we see our health as a service to others in the long run that we fully value its importance in our lives.

It comes as no surprise, therefore, that your average-Joe Kantian Fitlosopher is far more likely to see a lifestyle change in for the long haul. Gone are the chances of fleeting whims or ephemeral resolutions, and in their place lies resolute, universal rules for themselves and how they wish to live, much akin to how Kant believed we should navigate the maddening maelstrom that is general society.

But, wait. Is there a chance you could get . . . too Kant? Too boring?

Like with any of the philosophers inculcated into this series, there's a catch to Kant's stalwart nature to all things morality and ethics. First thing's first: Kant can be guilty of using the **naturalistic fallacy**, especially when trying to outline the notion of sacred rationality and consciousness in humans. A naturalistic fallacy basically suggests that anything that is defined as factually "natural" equates it with being good—the paleo diet, for example, espouses many examples of this logical incoherency. Avocados might be great and might be a plant, but I'll be damned if you start eating ten a day and not expect any weight change.

Experience on its own, some may argue, cannot be the sole factor that defines whether or not a thing can be moral. We gain no precise knowledge of morality from said experience; in a nutshell, we are unable to derive what something *ought* to be based purely on the arrangement of our conscious experience.

Of course, we could go into inextricable, arguably painful (at least for you lot) detail regarding the fallacies in Kant's argument.

But the important—and probably, much more relevant—details to include here are the effect on how one marries importance and duty with exciting real-life stuff, like spontaneous dinners and cosy Netflix binges with loved ones and skipping a gym session just *because* your body isn't feeling it.

Much fun has been poked at Kant for, lacking a better term, his old-before-his-years lifestyle. Basically, he was a boring old sod before boring old sods were given the liberty to act in such a way. Now, that was back in the time when he was alive. A time when you didn't have iPhones or ubiquitous rooftop bars popping up in every southwest area of London imaginable.

Sure, secret orgies would've probably been a thing, but you don't need to be Immanuel Kant to give those a miss.

So imagine having to be so attached to routine now, in a culture when moments of emotion and spontaneity often colour the sky-scraper-grey life is amassed with.

Having fun is no trivial pursuit.

The notion of play, and playing for its own sake, has had its revival in contemporary psychology. What was once deemed a feature of hedonism and seen as a method of respite, descale, or even indulgence is now considered a higher-tiered framework for creativity and improved health.

Play does not necessarily equate to a heavy night on the town or countless romantic conquests across the span of one's adulthood. Rather, play implies being one with the moment, all self-consciousness shed and revelling in the sheer lightness of living.

Defining "play" as a term has perplexed both philosophers and psychologists alike throughout the years. After all, how does one conceptualise the term "play," or view it in light of function and operation? Should play have a purpose? Can activities with a set objective even be considered part of the "play spectrum"?

The Play Spectrum is a concept that has been explored in an attempt to marry empirical support and that intuitive wisdom we feel from deep within. We *know* the feeling of a sunset's buttery light against our face and experience intangible, immaterial emotions in the face of such beauty. We *know* the experience of a baby's titter leaves us at the mercy of unconditional joy and a profound warmth for the timeline of human life. These are concepts imprinted deep within our bodies, widows that transcend experimental methodology and peer-reviewed studies. In order to further explore this human mystery, however, we do need to marry the esoteric with the empirical.

A Kantian Fitlosopher may at times disregard this innate sense of awe (ironically, given the OG philosopher's transcendental views) in favour of duty to themselves and thus others. One of the main things that might appear disparaging to Kantian Fitlosophers is that play is generally characterised as something marked by means rather than ends. In other words, the activity itself becomes more important than the end result. Nobody goes and builds sandcastles on the beach or thrusts themselves into December's snowy down, snow angels clustered everywhere, with the intention of strengthening neural connections or become better disciplined in the long run. We can easily, however, look at the overarching benefits of said means in a way that satisfies the values system of a Kantian Fitlosopher. Now might be wise to look at some of the science on the nature of play in order to convince you to put down the calorie tracker in favour of a spontaneous night on the town with your partner.

How can a Kantian Fitlosopher work hard but also play hard?

Welp, sometimes you gotta play fire with fire and try and twist your arm into thinking that playing can result in better work.

A statement from the paper by Zosh et al. (2018) exhibits the benefits of carving out spontaneity and play. Indeed, this research proposes the notion of a Play Spectrum to better define such a broad term. Kantian Fitlosophers might do well to consider the different nuances of play if this is something they genuinely struggle to fit into their lifestyle guilt-free.

Joy, or positive affect, has been linked to increased executive functions and academic outcomes (see Diamond, 2014 for a review) and even brain flexibility (Betzel et al., 2017). Iteration, or the mindful construction of new knowledge based on hypothesis testing and revising one's own knowledge over time, is a hallmark of learning and play (Piaget, 1962). Each of these characteristics is supported by the learning literature and is inherent in playful learning contexts.

In this instance, it might be worth taking up a hobby beyond fitness (unless, of course, a desirable sport is involved). When our brains are focused on certain activity to the point whereby background quirks fade or melt into obsequious blemishes on our consciousness—that sweet spot of «flow," one might say—it becomes a kind of distraction tool in that we forget our anxieties, woes, or heavy thoughts that may be holding us back from full concentration in our daily tasks.

All to say: by acknowledging that spontaneity, play, and joyful moments that cannot necessarily be explained by the constraints of duty or specific ends actually help us become the people we want to be, it becomes much easier to slide in that cake slice or last-minute trip abroad, knowing that some of the best things life can offer us aren't always found in dusty tomes or Fitbit trackers.

Duties can, if not careful, feel like a ball and chain, preventing us from soaring and exploring and seeing who we want to be, what lives we want to lead. Kantian Fitlosophers are diligent and hard-working, but at times it's worth checking in to see if the goals you are currently pursuing are, at their heart, truly the aims you feel are worth chasing down. It's very much worth taking a leap of faith, embracing glimpses of boundless, terrifying freedom, and seeing if any other duties might best appeal to our personal values out there.

FINDING YOUR FITLOSOPHY

After sifting through this deluge of options, there's every chance you might be feeling overwhelmed or confused rather than comforted. If that's the case, then consider this feeling your welcome party to philosophy. Spoiler alert: it doesn't get much easier from here on out. Joking aside, there's a reason I wanted to create a very basic overview of just a few famed thinkers from throughout history. One, to hopefully reveal the practical elements contained within the dusty tomes of philosophical thought. Hopefully now that you've read this book, you can see there are merits to discussing such thrilling topics as lying or whether or not truth is subjective. And two, basic frameworks create less overwhelm in the face of understanding ourselves. We don't need to analyse ourselves to the point of over-intellectualising; why trigger the torturous cycle of rumination and despair? We want to take the good bits of philosophy, not the anxiety-inducing aspects, thank you very much. Research indicates that if we orientate our constantly living toward "why do I do this," we actually don't get to the crux of solution-based living. It's much more fruitful to ask "what": what can I do right now to be better? What can I do at this moment to fulfill my needs? What are the required actions to develop a better version of myself?

Hence why *Fitlosophy* focuses solely on a select list of thinkers. We'd be here until the end of time if we took a more scenic route—and even then, some philosophers could even argue there'd be more of a time-like zeitgeist well beyond that idiom. Psychological research attempts to condense human personality insofar that we gain a better understanding of our own behaviours and how to change them. As a primary example, the factor-five model of personality is famed for the way it approaches understanding personality. Getting a base overview of your likes, dislikes, and behaviours in specific situations appears much more palatable when siphoned down into clear-cut categories. This was very much an element I tried to take into consideration when writing this book. Nobody needs to know the intricate details of David Chalmers' view on consciousness when there are, frankly put, more practical elements of the subject to be salvaged. And I say that with all the love in my heart for the subject matter that is consciousness and free will.

There are five traits described in the factor-five model as a means to explain human personality. These are Openness, Conscientiousness, Extroversion, Agreeableness, and Neuroticism. Researchers who are proponents of this model suggest human personality can be accounted for using these five traits. In recent years, some (fair and rounded) criticism has been expressed toward this approach: for one, it focuses primarily on Western-centric cultures, which means sampling bias might affect the way we interpret or understand how a person's behaviour reflects their internal world. Second, having five traits cover varying facets of personality seems somewhat underwhelming! They're currently thinking about tagging on another trait to make it the factor-six, supposedly. Whilst this is still meagre portioning, it's a step in the right direction—despite retaining that rather One Direction-esque name as its title.

The factor-five model was created in the sixties and has emerged as one of the less-empirically scathed personality analyses out there. (As much as I'm giving some side-eye to the Myers-Briggs test, if it helps people uncover more about themselves or encourage them to potentially grow, then I harbour no ill-feeling toward it.) Attempting to understand ourselves has its tendrils in major societal cornerstones, ranging from workplace settings all the way to dating app bios. These tend to manifest themselves under the guises of hotly pursued cultural tropes, such as horoscopes or enneagram profiles. Though not nearly as scientific as an independently researched personality model, it shares the underpinning drive that has possibly caused such demand for psychologists to explore this area of our lives: attaining certainty in an unpredictable world. If we know who we are, how we behave, what we are like in certain situations, and our motivational drivers, we feel better secured to take some security in our everyday lives. This book aims to provide you with profiles that might best fit you and your approaches to habit change in an effort to make your lifestyle goals more attainable. When we better understand ourselves, we are in a stronger position to make empowering choices for a future self that is best served by our habits in the now. So there might be some sense knowing whether you're a "total Virgo" now, after all.

One bone I have to contend with these personality models—and one which I hope has been at least subtly attended to in the book—is its lack of fluidity. The human tendency to label and categorise is useful in parts but can induce psychological rigidity if we're not careful. It doesn't matter how high your neuroticism levels are; odds are they'll go up if you're forced to attend a stressful job interview or first date with a beautiful person. Yet this should not define one's overall outlook or worldview. Similarly, just because you might have a more stringent attitude to exercise and diet for one period of your life doesn't mean you align your views with a Nietzschean Fitlosopher forevermore, let's take as an example. It might be that more will and drive is required for a sporting event but not for everyday living. Therefore, the beauty in understanding these varying philosophical approaches is that we can all learn from them. There will likely be a preference or inclination toward a certain approach that is personal to you. Equally, there exists a pragmatic concept in exploring and learning new ideas: to expand one's emotional toolkit should one way of acting no longer serve you at any given moment. Learning by sharing ideas is a powerful weapon in our arsenal of living out our lives as human beings.

And there's something irrevocably moving about learning through others. Over the years, I have seen many an individual achieve great things; achieving through means that I would have never considered to be my approach of choice. It's a given that I've learnt more from my clients than they from my own teachings, or at least, that's how I feel. In part, it was my clients who inspired me to write this. Secondly, I saw the pragmatic aspects of philosophy being dismissed all too readily by the scientific community. In fact, the parallels between habit change and philosophical worldviews became clearer to me as time wore on. One of the reasonings behind this book was based upon both my experience as both a coach and being an avid lover of all things psychology and philosophy. In truth, as much as we can tease and torment those despair-addled thinkers for looking at a coffee table and crying out at its existence, we have to concede something: they were on to a trick when it came to understanding and exploring the human condition.

There might've been moments when you skim read this book and thought, *well, I don't belong to any of these processes.* Reader, I implore you to consider this an exciting opportunity: a well of depth and riches to explore who you are and what makes you tick.

Sometimes, exercise can be a mere physiological process to help you dust away some cobwebs and get the heart rate up. I emphasise the "sometimes." More often than not, ask anyone, from the Olympian swimmer to the hobbyist judoka, and they'll describe the ways their movement instills their life with meaning. Human beings are storytellers, meaning-makers; we like to make ourselves seem a fanciful species by applying whimsy to our daily lives, right down to the last tea bag staining our kitchen surface. This book may hopefully induce an urge to find your why and explore the meaning behind exercise and lifestyle change. It could be as simple as seeing it in purely materialist terms, a la the Marxist Fitlosopher, or perhaps you might need to try on a few hats before you find one that best suits your own life. Life is about uncovering your values and seeing which approach behooves you the most. Values-based living is one way in which we can find out which motivational drivers connect to us the most. Is it aesthetics, performance, or play? Do we value hard work and tenacity, the climb to the top of our proverbial mountain, or finding purpose in the present? None are right and wrong; it's about finding intrinsic rulesets that help guide your actions. When you feel like you can stand back and examine the way you change your habits or approach exercise, you're in a better position to see which Fitlosophy suits you better.

Core values aren't tangible concepts like wealth or success. Though set values may help you, indirectly at least, carve out a path to reach these arbiters of happiness, they're not touchstones upon which you base your daily behaviour. Core values might look something like Honesty, Family, Empathy, Creativity, or Learning. We can figure out what makes us "tick" (or which values connect to us most at a given time) by reflecting on events in our lives that overwhelmed us with a sudden surge of meaning, of purpose. Was it when you felt true, deep happiness at a family Christmas event?

When you got promoted after years of slogging in a role? Or after having a truly profound conversation with a partner? It's worth having a think or even writing down these moments and the feelings experienced thereafter. They may provide vital clues in how you view your life or cultivate values.

This is where choosing our own personal values can help prevent us from becoming arseholes. Core values prevent people from playing the victimhood card. Rather than blaming their partner for not being able to fulfill their emotional needs after a bad day, an individual with core values understands and respects the need for separation and boundaries. They use their own values to understand what makes them tick, what will help get them out of that emotional funk. Values instill within us a yardstick to follow when life is at its toughest. That's why it's important to ask yourself these questions—to avoid finding yourself surrounded by manipulative arseholes or in situations that fail to make you grow or fulfill your sense of purpose.

- What is it the most that I value from my partner/colleague/ friend/family member?
- What kind of impact do I want to impart onto the world on a daily basis?
- What traits do I admire in successful people around me?
- What values represent your way of living (or aspired way of living)?
- In what ways in life can I be a little bit less of a douchebag?

Once you really start asking yourself what exactly that you value in life, you begin to get a clearer picture as to how to manifest all that good stuff in. Not by magical voodoo chanting and clutching amethyst crystals whilst feeding your fifteenth cat, mind you—through action. Take the courage to speak up more about your feelings if you value Honesty. Be less of a slob at work and make an effort to contribute to the team if you value Responsibility. You can dive straight in, or if you feel as if you need to visualise your values a bit more and see which direction to go in, make a similar table to the one below and begin to identify your perceived values that need a bit more supporting and growth. Visually speaking, it might give you the kick up the bum to actually live your values and not live your life through a narcissistic eggshell. The lower the score, the more actions you will need to implement.

Finding Fitlosophies that most suit you will involve digging into what you value the most out of life. Is it joy, new experiences, or routine? Is it having a set moral guide that allows you to behave in a specific way? The only way, in my opinion, we can best understand ourselves is by looking at the things we value the most. And if our actions aren't in alignment with the values we set ourselves, unsurprisingly this feels fairly crappy. We might feel lost, purposeless like we're not quite sure what to do with ourselves or that there's something missing from our lives. That's because there are: actions that align with what we stand for. In instances such as these, there's likely something deeper going on, like a misjudgment of what we value or even a shift in what we hold dear. All of these (and much more) are part of the painfully beautiful journey held within humanity. In short, we can only determine the approach that matters to us most based on our core values—which tend to proliferate across our life in a much more general way.

How you view exercise and lifestyle change impinges on a multitude of factors. And whilst this book can't necessarily answer that for you, what it hopefully might instill is a need, an urge to explore who you are at a fundamental level. Asking yourself what fulfills you and what gives you meaning—even if, like the Postmodernist, that might be a transient gesture in of itself—might not solve the uncertainty that life holds, but it can offer you a solid foundation for undertaking the actions that best suit you and you alone. This is the magical albeit downright frustration aspect of philosophy: there's no right answer, not really. Only valid and sound arguments. Some arguments—and premises, for that matter—might be, objectively speaking, better put together than others, but ultimately the both of you are still debating as to whether or not Mary knows what red or green is after spending a lifetime cooped away in a black-and-white room.

There is no right answer, not really. Only one that is right for you. One that works for your lifestyle, core values, and goals at heart. And if that approach suddenly feels stilted one day or acts more like a nagging partner holding you back? Well, dear reader, there's plenty more Fitlosophy to explore, sink your teeth into, and try your hand at. Movement is meant to work with our lives, not against it.

That's one solid philosophy, I think, that we can all agree on.

ABOUT THE AUTHOR

Sophie's love for philosophy began as a teenager. She studied the topic extensively in an autonomous fashion, eventually using it as a fundamental methodology for her approach to life coaching. She is now finishing up her MSc in psychology whilst training clients both on and offline.

What does an author stand to gain by asking for reader feedback? A lot. In fact, it's so important in the publishing world that they've coined a catchy name for it: "social proof." And without social proof, an author may as well be invisible in this age of digital media sharing.

So if you've enjoyed *Fitlosophy*, please consider giving it some visibility by reviewing it on the sales platform of your choice. Your honest opinion could help potential readers decide whether or not they would enjoy this book too.

Made in the USA
Middletown, DE
10 January 2022

57603539R00097